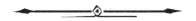

ISBN 978-0-483-55092-6
PIBN 10786005

This book is a reproduction of an important historical work. Forgotten Books uses state-of-the-art technology to digitally reconstruct the work, preserving the original format whilst repairing imperfections present in the aged copy. In rare cases, an imperfection in the original, such as a blemish or missing page, may be replicated in our edition. We do, however, repair the vast majority of imperfections successfully; any imperfections that remain are intentionally left to preserve the state of such historical works.

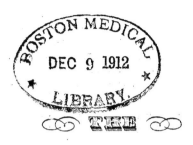
THE

IOWA CATLIN.

1278

A JOURNAL OF

MEDICINE & SURGERY.

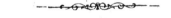

ORIGINAL COMMUNICATION.

HOG CHOLERA.

The disease among swine known as hog cholera, has, by scientific men been positively demonstrated to be, *Trichinosis*, caused by reception of *Trichinæ Spiralis* into the alimentary canal, by eating raw flesh infested with the parasite, encysted in the flesh eaten. In process of digestion, the *trichinæ* are liberated from the cyst, and are rapidly developed sexually, and by propagation of their species, multiply to billions. In a short time they migrate from the alimentary canal toward the surface of the body. As they pass through the tissues, the irritation (or damage done) consequent upon their piercing the walls of the stomach and intestines, we have the manifestation of the disease known as hog cholera, viz: retching and vometing, with choleraic discharges from the bowels, which evidence the great irritability of the digestive track, and which can be readily understood by observing the damage done to the alimentary canal, by reason of the passage of millions of the parasite to the square inch. Later we have indisposition to exertion, muscular soreness amounting to painful muscular rheumatism, with inability to use the muscles of the jaw to masticate food. After a certain time, if the infection be slight, the parasite becomes encapsulated in the muscular tissue; the grave symptoms subside; the animal recovers, and so far as this particular animal will be concerned, may have continual good health thereafter.

The *trichina* is developed from the ovum of the tape-worm, (*Tœnia mediocanellata*,) of which, rats and mice find cast-off joints in privy vaults; or domestic fowls may find them in human excrement scattered about on the surface of the ground. The ovum of the tape-worm eaten by the rat, or domestic fowl, develop *cisticerci*. The hog feeding upon rats or chickens infested with *cisticerci* develop *trichinosis*, or hog cholera.

A hog having recovered from *trichinosis*, may grow to the proportion and appearance of a fine porker, though his muscular structure contain millions of encysted *trichinæ* to the cubic inch. In this state they have ceased to be disturbers of the health. If this recovered *trichinous* animal die, and a herd of swine are permitted to feast upon the carcass, each animal partaking of the flesh will be infected with *trichinæ*, (hog cholera,) and each animal so infected will infect other healthy swine through the medium of the excreta from the infected animal, and thus it will be seen, that swine raisers have the elements of hog cholera constantly in their midst, and for want of a proper understanding of the nature and cause of the disease, are in danger of infecting their entire herd of swine, as well as many of the human family.

Since there are no remedies which will destroy the parasite, without at the same time destroying the infected animal; or in the least counteract or modify the infection of *trichinæ*, (hog cholera,) hog breeders should direct their attention to police and hygienic regulation which should extend over the premises. The hog stable and pasture should be remote from the hennery or haunts of domestic fowls. Dogs and cats should not be permitted within the inclosure occupied by swine. The water supply should not be in close proximity to privies, as the water seepage from such vaults might contaminate the water, and be a medium through which infection take place. The carcasses of all dead animals should at once be buried in deep pits remote from the water supply, or carted off to the soap factory. Hog stables should be isolated from other farm buildings containing grain, or which furnish harbors for rats. It should be constructed in such manner that rats could not find an entrance under its floor. In case infection enters your herd, the well swine should be removed to other lots. Do not be satisfied with throwing out diseased swine as cases occur; if you do, you leave behind material in excreta from the infected animal which will be devoured by the healthy swine left in the infected pen.

All useless animals of the dog or cat kind should be disposed of, as they are parasitic breeders, and easily infect other animals when in close proximity.

Finally, swine infested with *trichinosis*, (hog cholera) should be killed at once, and only be used for making soap, as their flesh will never be fit food for man or animal. As a glandered horse is by law condemned to death as a hygienic measure to prevent the spread of the *glander contagium*; for the same reason the cholera hog should be declared a nuisance, and be abated.

This article was not written with the view of exhausting the subject, but simply to state positive facts, which can be easily demonstrated; and also to show the great need of an Iowa State Board of Health whose duty it should be, to investigate any and all causes of disease which may compromise the health of, or endanger the lives of the people.

E. LAWRENCE, M. D.

Deemed of public inportance, this article was first published in the Osceola New Era.

MEDICAL LITERATURE.

Article I. Surgical Clinic. Is Carcinoma of the Blood, or is it a Local Affection? Scirrus of the Breast. Operation for; how and when to perform Excision.

By W. W. DAWSON, M. D.,
Surgeon to Good Samaritan Hospital, Cincinnati, O.

Gentlemen:--Scirrus of the breast, a disease so frequent and destroying so many valuble lives, challenges our study and presents claims upon the best recources of our profession. It is most usually found in women 'from thirty years to fifty years of age, occasionally it attacks the young, and is by no means uncommon in the old; three-score and ten is not an exemption. About five years ago I operated on a married lady, aged 20, for a rapidly developed scirrus of the left mamma. The peri-glandular fat was freely infiltrated with indurated masses, these I removed as completely as possible; since the excision she has given birth to a child; there has been no recurrence of the disease. My oldest patient was 60; a few months after the operation the affection reappeared.

The years after the climacteric seems to be the fated ones for the development of malignant disease. The dangers consequent upon child-bearing having passed, good health and long life seeming to be assured, all is suddenly arrested by the appearance of a tumor in the breast. sometimes it has been heralded by pain, but more often it has attained consid.

erable size before its presence is discovered. Yesterday I examined a lady who had a scirrus growth in the left breast as large as an orange; some months ago she detected it when bathing; it was at that time at least one inch in diameter, but it had given her no pain whatever—and now, although the tumor be so large, her sufferings are more mental than phys· ical. Pain, when present, as an element of diagnosis in malignant degenernation of the mammary gland cannot be relied on, as it has no definite character: in some instances it is of a burning stinging nature, in others it is described as if needles were being thrust into the tumor. Again, some patients complain of dull aching sensations in both the affected and unaffected part of the organ.

The retracted nipple and stone-like tumor are the two factors of most value, the first, like the skin dimples, produced by a fibrous prolongation from the tumor, is almost always present, the last must be recognised for an unquestioned definition of the case.

In the patient which I present to-day, and the same was true in the woman upon whom I operated two weeks ago, the pain is of the dull aching character, the nipple is retracted and the tumor has the phathognhomonic hardness.

Amputation of the breast for malignant disease has justly been regarded as an unpromising operation. Recurrence of the disease has been the rule, and exceptions to this rule having been so few some surgeons have hesitated—have doubted the propriety of a resort to the knife.

Is there a period in the history of carcinoma of the breast when the disease is essentially local. Or is it always but one of a number of expressions of a cancerous cachexia. The promise of an operation depends upon the solution to this question. If the first part of the question be answered in the affirmative then there can be no doubt upon the propriety of a resort to the knife, if however, the latter be affirmed, then we may well hesitate upon adopting operative interference.

The observation of most practitioners affirm the proposition that there is a period in most cases when the disease is confined to the locality—in fact to the tumor itself. The clinical experience of operating surgeons furnishes cases that ought to be accepted as conclusive upon this matter. The cases of Sir James Paget, in which his patient lived eleven years and a half after the removal of a scirrus breast and died of muscular atrophy, presents evidence of much weight and goes far towards establishing the affirmation of the proposition. Case books abound in such instances but it must however be admitted that the unfortunate out-number the fortunate. The number of those in which the disease did not reappear is less than those in which there was a recurrence. The reason of this will be apparant in the settlement of the question as to whether the disease originates in the tumor or rather whether the tumor is the disease or only an expression of a vice in the blood.

The successful cases in which the knife has been early resorted to, goes far toward determining as I have said the local origin of the disease.

Pathologists upon this subject differ radically, their teachings are scarcely so uniform as are the experiences of operators.

Sir James Paget says: "I would say that a cancer is from the first both a constitutional and a specific disease. I believe it to be constitutional, in the sense of having its origin and chief support in the blood, by which the constitution of the whole body is maintained; and I believe it to be specific. 1st, in the sense of its being dependent on some specific material, which is different from all the natural constituents of the body, and different from all the material formed in other processes of disease, and 2nd, in the sense of its presenting in the large majority of cases structures which are specific or peculiar, both in their form and in their mode of life."

Such an assertion, so emphatic upon the blood theory of the disease may well cause a pause in the enthusiastic surgeon, but when it is placed by the side of the following more recent and equally authoritative statement it loses somewhat of its force and takes the position of advice rather than of command; of opinion, rather than law. Billroth in his Surgical Pathology says. "We may say that Carcinomatæ are very infectious tumors, and that this infection which first attacks the lymphatic glands, afterwards more distant, organs is probably due to the passage of elements from the tumor (whether of cells or juice is not yet known) through the lymph vessels and veins into the blood." Here the local origin of cancer is clearly stated; forciby taught. It cannot be denied that there is in some instances a true cancerous cahexia, and that the disease is occasionally hereditary, but these facts do not prove that it is always constitutional, always primarily in the blood. Allow me to state a few significant points, and I beg, gentlemen, your close attention to them.

(1) A recurrence does not prove that a disease is in the system, for we find this disposition to return in a certain class of fibroids that have never been suspicioned of originating in the blood.

(2) In a great number of cases, scirrus of the breast is traced directly to a blow upon the organ. Previously, the woman had been in robust health, yet a malignant tumor followed a slight trauma. Cancer of the lip is often traced directly to the irritation of the pipe-stem.

(3) After removal, in fact often during the course of the disease, the general health of the patient is good.

(4) When the disease returns, it is usually in the cicatrix or in its neighborhood.

(5) A cancerous tumor may exist for years and no dyscrasia be manifested.

(6) The truly impressive fact that the excision of unquestioned cancerous tumors, patients have lived for years in a state of *positive health.*

(7) Virchow teaches that, in many cases, cancer is of local origin, and the researches of pathologists of the present day tend to the verification of

the views of this great and original investigato.:

Assuming then with Billroth, Virchow and others that scirrus of the breast is for a time at least, in numerous cases local, we may well enquire why the operation for its removal has been so unfortunate, why the disease has so frequently returned.

Three reasons may be stated, (1) the operation is not performed sufficiently early while the disease is essentially confined to the gland, before the "passage of elements from whether of cells or juice through the lymphatic vessies and veins into the blood." The faulty plan of removing only the tumor, not excising the unaffected part of the gland and the neighboring fat, in both of which there may be out-liers of malignant matter not perceptible to the eye. Upon this subject Sir James Paget says: "The existence of cancer cells infiltrated amongst the tissues which surround the actual cancerous tumor, and which to the naked eye may appear to be perfectly healthy, has however now been domonstrated by more than one pathologist." (3) The disease usually reappears in the cicatrix, hence the entire skin with the tumor and gland should be removed, leaving an open wound to heal by granulation. An effort is usually made to form a handsome looking operation by bringing the skin together. How often are hopes of union by the first intention realized? Seldom, I think will be the common answer; pockets of matter, on the contrary, have been the rule. As the flaps although united by sutures, in a few days recede, we might as well, if we had no other reason, leave, at the beginning, the floor of the wound exposed.

Why is the recurrence so frequent in the cicatrix? Billroth answers this question when he says that the mammary gland is "a derivative of the epidermis, a cutaneous fat-gland on a large scale." And that mammary cancer "seems to me always to begin with a coincident enlagement of the small round epithelial cells in the acini and with small-celled infiltration of the connective tissue around them." Here clinical experience is reinforced by pathological demonstrations.

Another weighty suggestion for removing the skin arising from the kinship between the mammary gland and epithelial tissue, is the fact that epithelial cancers, of unmistakable carcinomatous nature, when radically removed, do not show a recurrent disopsition.

The rule then should be,—*operate early, remove with the tumor the unaffected part of the gland, the peri-glandular fat and skin.*

Two weeks ago I amputated the left breast for scirrus, and today I bring before you another lady similarly affected and upon whom I propose to make the same operation. Whilst my patient is becoming anæsthetised I desire to call your attention to this wound now two weeks after the excision. You will remember that the amputation was made in the manner which I have just described, removing the entire mass down to the pectoral muscles; the wound filled with vasaline and over this placed a compress. My surgical iuterne, Dr. Samuels, informs me that there has scarcely been enough pus discharged to soil the lint. When the wound is uncovered you see how clean and healthy it looks, how rapidly it is contracting. In my experience I have seen no dressing equal to vasaline, it is essentially antiseptic, effectually excluding by its consistence the air.

But to return to the case before us. This lady is about fifty years of age, and first noticed an enlargement of the left breast about eight months ago; since then the whole gland has rapidly enlarged until it is now more than twice its normal size. The induration is unequal, at one point it is hard, stone-like to the touch. The skin is firm, leathery, and its pores unusually large; there is no dimple upon it, nor does it pit on pressure. The tumor seems to be firmly fixed to the tissue beneath. The nipple has been retracted for three months. I can find no axillary involvement. Her general health is excellent. Is this a favorable case for an operation?

There are some unpromising features. (1) Its rapid development. (2) The extensive involvement of the skin. (3) Its close attachment to the pectoral muscles.

An operation, the entire excision of the gland, and the skin covering it offers her all that there is in the resources of our art.

Internal remedies have proved useless. Compression has ended only in disappointment. Caustics are barbarous. Some of you may remember, how, a few years ago, the hopes of the affected were raised, only to be cast down, by cundurango. It was championed by unscrupulous doctors, and certified to by soulless politicians. Thousands were spent for it and in no single instance did it give comfort, much less affect a cure.

Will a thorough excision, even should recurrence take place, prolong life? I think both pahthologist and clinicians would answer this question in the affirmative aud upon a proposion closely associated, both classes would also affirm, that the removal adds to the comfort of the patient.

With two or three bold sweeps of the knife I remove the whole mass, the skin, the gland enclosing the scirrus and a portion of fat. The large part of the neighboring fat still remains, this I dissect out with the forceps and curved scissars.

I regret to see that the scirrus tumor had already seized the pectoral muscles, an unfavorable complication always. Acting upon the hope that the disease may yet be local, confined to the gland and its immediate neighbors, I think it best to pick up the affected parts of the muscle and divede them freely—below—deeper than the infiltration seems to extend.

Now let us examine the tumor. I make a section through the most solid part, its consistence is cartilage like. The cut surface has a greyish appearace. with here and there a greyish stria, and yields when scraped a fluid a little more dense than water. The hard character of the tumor however settles its nature, no other morbid product equals scirrus in this quality.

Unpromising as this case is in many of its features I have however, no doubt but the operation if it does not comple tely relieve will prolong this woman's life and add to her comfort.

More than 18 months ago I was called to Kentucky to operate on a case of scirrus of the breast. I found the gland hard, boulder-like and an ulcerated surface upon its summit 2 inches by 1½ inches in extent. I was about to decline the case, it was so unpromising, when it occurred to me.to remove the mass, according to the plan I have discussed. She is now in robust health. In an effort to make a handsome looking operation, the skin, with cancer germs, would have been left and my patient in all probability would ere this have been destroyed. I can call to mind a number of operations in which I committed this error, that is, I saved skin that was not above suspicion, so that I could close the wound according to the instructions of the books. Gant, after advising that the lips of the wound be brought together says; "Primary union somtimes takes place in a few days; but more frequently this union is spurious, and the wound opens up partially at least, with suppuration, and heals by granulation."

Erichsen thinks union by primary adhesion more frequent, but admits when discussing the two plans that recurrence most usually takes place in the cicatrix and suggests (an important suggestion by the way), that cancer cells may be eliminated by the suppuration process.

If then, as Gant observes, the flap fall, in most instances, apart, and as Erichsen asserts in the suppurative process cancer germs, may be destroyed, healing by granulation is an end rather to be sought than avoided.

As I do not intend to bring the lips of the wound together it matters little in what direction the incisions are made, whether vertically, from side to side or in the course of the pectoralis major.

I would again, gentlemen, repeat that in estimating tumors of the breast one thing you should never lose sight of—I mean the peculiar hardness of scirrus. It cannot be likened to any other morbid growth. It is nowhere else seen except in the base of an epithelial ulcer. This hardness characterizes the tumor in all stages of its growth, it may be detected as well in the deposits the size of a filbert, as in that which has attained the dimensions of the closed hand.

A question sometimes arises, and we are called upon to decide between the solidity of a fibroid and the hardness of a scirrus, the first is elastic, the last unyielding.

When it is remembered that the large majority of tumors of the mammæ are malignant, most of them being scirrus, a few encephaloid, still fewer colloid and occasionally a sarcomata, it would be a safe rule to follow to remove all having a suspicion of cancerous degeneration. If the tumor prove to be benign, one breast is left which is sufficient for maternity, if it be cancerous you have given your patient all the advatages of an early and radical operation.—*Cincinnatti Lancet and Observer.*

Relation of the Sense of Hearing to Voice and Speech, as regards deaf Mutes.

BY J. R. DAVY. M. D., Cincinnati, Ohio.

Professor Dungleson in his lectures in Jefferson Medical College used to teach that the voice depended so greatly on the sense of hearing that when the latter was lost, the former speedily disappeared. Thus the fact that dumbness is the general companion of deafness was thought by him to be strictly unavoidable inasmuch as the individual having lost the faculty of audition, possessed nothing by which to measure and modulate his voice. In this condition of disease the muscles of the larynx became gradually weaker until at the end of a certain period, the voice was irretrievably lost.

This idea of Prof. Dungleson was in accordance with the teachings of the day; that it was to a great extent ill-founded, will appear when we have critically examined the subject.

Cophosis or deafness is an impaired condition of the apparatus of audition;

We have evidence that the brain proper of a deaf-mute is affected or that the faculty of hearing, assuming there is one, is at all abnormal beyond being in a rudimentary condition. In a well nourished individual we must conclude that the organ for appreciating sound wave is, with this exception in fact no matter how the so-called apparatus of audition, whose office is to transform units of matter into units of mind, is distorted.

A very important yet perplexing question is—where does the receiving apparatus end and the appreciating apparatus begin? It is highly supposable that there is a chain of nervous matter passing on from the fourth ventricle to some restricted portion of the cerebrum; but when we have followed the auditory nerve from the membranous labyrinth of the internal ear to the gray nucleus in the floor of the fourth ventricle, we have our say in the matter—the rest is mere speculation.

The term appreciation, applied by writers to the function of the rods of Corti, is, I think, a misapplication since it might be interpreted to imply intelligence, an impossibility so far away from the great central organ.

The rods of Corti may vibrate in unison with the different tones, but the impressions arising from these vibrations, must be carried inward to the brain and their character arrive there. We may say this much with truth—the receiving part of the auditory apparatus lies external to the Portio Mollis of the 7th pair, and the appreciating part, as absolute in existence without being understood by us, lies internal to that nerve.

The books tell us that destruction of the Membrana Tympani does not produce deafness, the vibration of sound, and even of musical tones still being recognised by the internal ear. This latter comprising the cochlea, vestibule and semi-circular canals (of which the cochlea performs the most important part), is where the nervous element begins, and where, unfortunately, our knowledge ceases. It is not necessary to say that most cases of deafness depend upon some fault of the internal ear.

The voice is ascribed by physiologists to the vibration of the true vocal cords assisted to some extent by the trachea, and the resonant cavities of the larynx and mouth. The intrinsic muscles of the larynx control the apparatus, and keep it in tune, as it were. These little muscles are supplied by filaments derived from the spinal accessory through the communicating branch to the pneumogastric, and are under the control of the will, though like other voluntary muscles, act in obedience to another control when the will is absent.

The characters of the voice have been enumerated as intensity, quality, and pitch. Pitch depends upon the length and tension of the vocal cords. Quality of tone differs with different sexes, the child, and the adult; and even different individuals of the same age and sex. Intensity is the result of forced action of the apparatus.

What concerns us more particularly in this connection is the faculty of language. Words are composed of certain characters which represent sounds. These are called vowels and consonants. The former are produced by the vocal cords, and the latter by the combined action of the larynx and mouth—they are divided further into palatals, linguals, labials, gutturals and nasals. To produce a certain sound we must bring a certain set of muscles into action. If it be the sound of one of our own words, we pronounce it with ease and fluency; if a foreign sound, it is pronounced with difficulty. Every adult who has studied a foreign language knows with what trouble he has learned to speak it. In the individual of one language, the muscles, so to speak, have formed a bed for themselves in which they play, producing the requisite degree of change in the organ to make the normal sounds, and no more. In another tongue the sounds are different, requiring an additional or different action of the laryngeal muscles.

A new born child may be compared with a deaf-mute so far as the condition of the larynx is concerned. The muscles of each are simply undeveloped, and may be brought out by proper training; while the noises produced by both are the result of an almost passive condition of the larynx; hardly deserving the name of voice.

The importance of educating these muscles in the deaf-mute will be seen at once. But in this we will have a greater difficulty to contend with than in the young child. The child gets almost every idea leading to the production of voice through the ear, whose use the other is deprived of.

This brings us to consider the very important question as to whether or not deaf-mutes are sensible of speaking audibly, and if so how do they receive such impressions. But before I answer these questions I wish to relate my experience at the "Taubstummen Anstalt" of Vienna. At the "K. K. Taubstummen Anstalt, of Vienna, deaf and dumb children are taught to speak "viva voce," and not with signs as is the usual method in this country and France.

I was fortunate enough to be present at a public examination of the pupils of this institution. The pupils with whom the affection was mostly congenital, were from eight to fourteen years of age; and those farthest advanced had been in the institution about four years. The first boy called up had been a hydrocephalic child. He looked instantly at the mouth of the instructor pronouncing each word over after him with a peculiar snoring sound yet distinctly enough to be understood. The next was a bright little fellow (affection congenital) who caught the question quickly, and answered them readily and distinctly. With this boy quite a number of tests were given. The teacher wrote something on a slate, and handed it to me. Then going through the motions that it would require to utter it without making the slightest sound, the boy understood and replied immediately. I then tried the same thing myself with a similar result.

The boy was then placed with his back to the teacher and class, and questions were given him in a very loud voice. He exhibited no signs of hearing them, but turned around suddenly after a knock on the floor. He was again placed in the same position, and told to remain until he was called. In about a half minute he turned around imagining something had been said when no one had uttered a word. There was some difficulty making this boy understand the English sound T. He invariably called it D. After several fruitless attempts in the ordinary way, the instructor seized the boy's hand, and, pronouncing the latter against its posterior surface, succeeded at once in conveying the idea.

After this, others, male and female, were introduced talking fluently and without effort; yet absolutely devoid of all sense of hearing, and he had been born so. They all spoke in a peculiar singing monotone, which I took as additional evidence of complete deafness.

I have recently had conversation with Mr. Middleton, of this city who has had thirty-six years experience as an instructor in deaf and dumb institutions in this country. He informed me that often while playing upon a musical instrument the pupils would come up and touch the instrument with the finger, and express themselves as pleased with the impressions they received. When a band was playing in the street they would lay their hands on the window pane, and seemingly enjoy it.

We can now return to the question "are deaf-mutes sensible of speaking audibly?"

After my experience at the Vienna *Taubstummen Anstalt,* I have no hesitancy in answering yes. To determine the extent of this knowledge and the precise manner of acquiring it, is exceedingly difficult. If we take the ideas of writers on the subject, we will say that the impression of sound reaches them in only two ways—through vibrations of the air, and vibrations of the cranial bones.

Dalton denies the existence of the last, except to the slightest extent; for, says he, were this the case we could hear the sounds of our heart an l lungs. It is unreasonable to suppose that they receive impressions of sound in the usual way—_i. e._, through the vibrations of the air. They must get such impressions then through the vibrations of the solid tissues repeated until they reach the internal ear. But we cannot explain in this way all the phenomena peculiar to deaf-mutes. When the instructor whispers against the back of the pupil's hand the vibrations of that whisper, were certainly, not continued as far as the internal ear with sufficient force to be perceived. It is possible that the nerves of common sensation have something to do with this, yet it would be hasty in me to make such an assertion without knowing the importance of the phenomenon above referred to. The deaf mute feels however, that muscles are contracting, air is rushing through the passages, and vibrations are going on; and according to the quality and extent of the impressions received in this way, is his knowledge of speaking audibly. The seeming paradox of "deafness without dumbness" is by this explaine l at once; an l it does not seem impossible, that by education the so-called deaf-mute may eventually be made to modulate his voice.

The fact that the internal laryngeal muscles are under the control of the will; and that the individual is sensible of bringing them into action, makes the truth of the last assertion more apparent

With these facts in our minds we cannot fail to see that the only proper treatment for dumbness is education of the vocal muscles. By the proper training muscles may be developed in the leg or arm of any individual; and why not in the larynx? The larynx of a congenital deaf-mute is supplied with muscles like that of any other child, and these muscles possess the same susceptibility to education, only the manner of causing them to act properly is difficult. In the complete loss of function of the ear, the sense of hearing may be imperfectly replaced by the touch or sight; and these, one or both, might be used in teaching the congenital deaf-mute to articulate. By the aid of the eye he can read the lips of the instructor, or with a mirror he can modify the position of his own mouth and larynx so far as to produce the necessary sounds. By the touch he can determine vibrations in any solid body, and moreover discriminate between sounds of different pitch. With the fingers pressed against the larynx almost any one can determine the difference in the sounds proceeding from that organ, and can we doubt that this is much more perfect in individuals whose tactile sensibility far surpasses ours.

It has been urged against the articulating method that life is too short to accomplish very much in this tedious way, and the amount of troul l far in excess of the good derived from it. I question the propriety of this

objection, as I believe that the present education modifies to a certain extent the existence of the trouble in coming generations.

Being outcasts from society, deaf mutes generally marry among themselves; and this, according to the laws of reproduction, tends to perpetuate the malady. If the articulate method is pursued the vocal organ may
be made to retain its power despite the continued inability of the ear; if
the sign method is used instead, the voice connot fail to perish after a certain period.

A recent work entitled "Deaf, not Dumb," by Mr. Ackers, of London;
has appeared, and of which, the British Medical Journal of Oct. 6th, has a
short review. Mr. Ackers has visited personally nearly all the deaf and
dumb institutions in Europe and America, and decides very positively in
favor of the articulate method; although he concludes that the French
system is more readily taught. The most fertile cause of total deafness
he sets down as intermarrying of the congenitally deaf—of the accidental
causes, scarlet fever is the most frequent.

In conclusion I will say this paper is presented simply to call attention
to some facts which are not generally understood. My attempt at a solution of the physiological problem, "Deafness without Dumbness," is by no
means offered as final or complete.

The fact to which special attention is directed, is that dumb children
may be taught to articulate whether their loss of speech arises from accidental or congenital deafness.— *Cincinnati Lancet and Observer.*

Nitrate of Pilocarpia,

The physiological action of the infusion of Jaborandi is so powerful and
clearly defined that it is astonishing how little its therapeutic value has
been turned to account. Nevertheless, it must be admitted that the
study of this energetic agent presents serious difficulties, from the fact
that its leaves are often adulterated, besides being frequently ill-preser-
ved as found in the markets.

The discovery and isolation of *pilocarpia,* the active principle of that
plant, will enable us, however, to arrive at the precise therapeutic indica-
tion of this drug; furthermore, the patient will no longer be nausiated
by the disagreeable taste of the infusion, nor can the different results be
attributed to a difference in the quality of the medicine.

In the present article we will confine ourselves to the physiological
effects produced by absorption of the alkaloid, and later refer to the conditions in which the practitioner should avail himself of this modifier of the
salivary and cutaneous secretions.

Our experiments were made at the *Hotel de Caen;* we used the *nitrate of pilocarpia* hypodermically, the dose being from two and a half centigram-mes (3-10 to 3-8 grs.),—this salt is very soluble, and is therefore readily adapted for this form of medication.

. .The observations were made upon six patients, five of whom had some slight surgical trouble, and the sixth, a young man, suffered from phthisis pulmonalis. The following are the phenomena which we observed; one or two minutes, at most, after the injection, the patient felt flushes of heat in the face and a smarting sensation in the lumbar region; his counten-ance colored and his eyes were injected; a moment later an abnormal se-cretion of saliva filled his mouth and caused him to spit for eight or ten second.s The saliva is clear, watery and usually tasteless; sometimes, however, it is mixed with an abundant expectoration.

At the end of three minutes, small drops of sweat appeared upon the alæ of the nose; the brow presented nearly the same phenomenon; finally diaphoresis became general and was sufficient to soil the mattress.

The thermometer placed in the axilla showed no elevation of tempera-rure, 98 3-5 to 99 deg. Fahrenheit. The pulse, on the contrary, was un-steady; in the space of ten minutes it rose to 140, only to fall in a quarter of an hour later to 75—generally, it varied from 95 to 110.

In one case the heart palpitated forcibly, yet no murmur was heard. Respiration was normal.

About ten minutes after injection, three of the patients felt a desire to urinate; in each case the urine was diminished in amount, and the act of micturation caused a burning sensation in the urethral canal.

In every case vision was more or less disturbed, lachrymation was pro-duced and sight was less distinct, objects appeared as though enveloped in a veil.

As respects hearing, there was a sensation of buzzing and ringing in the ears, with approaching deafness. The digestive apparatus, with its at-tachments, also showed signs of disturbance; the tongue was slighty swol-len and become painful at its base; there were nausia and vomiting. yet the latter was not abundant.

Thirty-five minutes after the appearance of the first phenamenon, the countenance was less flushed, the skin became cool, the extremeties were cold, the limbs itched and the pulse was weak.

The patients were scarcely able to walk; they staggered and would have fallen had they not supported themselves. The most feeble were com-pletely exhausted, and, showing signs of stupor, they rested with their heads inclined over a basin receiving the saliva which, without effort, flowed from their mouths in abundance. Such are the curious effects which appeared in the first forty-five minutes, then little by little the se-cretion of saliva decreased, the perspiration became less copious, there was less feelings of malaise, and finally, at the end of an hour or two, everything had ceased.

The mean quantity of saliva secreted by each patient was 500 grammes

(16 ounces), but in one case it even amounted to 900 grammes; the perspiration, sufficient to saturate both mattress and covers.

The following fact is also rather peculiar; a woman received an injection of 0,025 milligramme (2-5 gr. nearly) of nitrate of pilocarpia in the arm; the above symptoms all appeared and passed away, but in the evening she had a second attack of sweating and salivation as abundant as the first. A soldier presented this same peculiarity, yet more strikingly, for in this case did the attack not only re-appear in the evening, but also on the following morning, at an hour corresponding with the time of the injection on the day previous.

Such, then, are the physiological phenomena which we witnessed, and one can readily understand from the rapidity and certainty of action of this alkaloid, what position it will command in future therapeutics.—*L' Annee Medicale.*

Piles Treated with Carbolic Acid Injection— Radical Cure.

By A. B. Cook, A. M., M. D, Professor of the Science and Art of Surgery and Clinical Surgery, Kentucky School of Medicine; Professor of the Principles and Practice of Surgery, Louisville Medical College.

The purpose of this article is briefly to direct the attention of the Profession to the value of corbolic acid as a remedial agent in the radical cure of hæmorrhoids. The frequency of the disease and the great dread of patients generally to submit to any form of treatment which will subject them to a painful operation and confinement to bed for two or three weeks, induces me to mention this simple method, which, in the great majority of cases, will supersede the knife, ligature, nitric acid, and clamp, heretofore the usual remedies where there is considerable dilatation of the hæmorrhoidal veins. Patients, rather than submit to an operation, content themselves with the use of various cathartics, laxatives, and astringent and anodyne unguents, which, wihout effecting a cure, frequently give little or no relief. A temporising treatment, under which the disease is usually aggravated, and finally the victims, under the impression that the general practitioner of surgery does not understand the treatment of the case, or that it is too insignificant to elicit his special study, and attention, fall into the hands of advertising specialists, who promise a certain cure without the knife, ligature or caustic. The inconvenience and suffering caused by enlarged or inflamed hæmorrhoides, and the ready relief given, may be inferred from the following cases:

Mrs.————aged twenty-six; married six years; occupation seamstress, sewing on a machine; sanæmic; has for a long time been suffering from habitual constipation; she has had piles for ten years—her father and other members of the family having suffered in like manner—a hereditary disease; she had external and internal piles, which had been inflamed, and caused much suffering for months. The external, several in number, situated at the junction of the skin and mucous membrane, were of long standing, small, hard, projecting like vegetations and exceedingly sensitive; these were removed with the scissors; warm anodyne fomentations were ordered locally to allay the tenderness, and the following laxative: R.—Magnesiæ carb. oz ½; magnesiæ sulph., drachms 2., potassæ bitartrat, sulphur sublimed, aa oz ½. M. Ft. Pulv. S. a teaspoonful in half glass of water once or twice daily if necessary. The external trouble was relieved in a few days, but at each evacuation, or in the act of coughing, an inflamed hæmorrhoid would protrude and cause acute pain, to which I was called several times. For several days she declined to have anything done, assigning as a reason that a former physician who had treated her father advised her never to submit to an operation, as it would be dangerous. The laxatives, unguents, suppositories, etc., etc., having failed to give relief, and being assured that the operation was simple, without danger or much suffering, and that it would give speedy relief, she consented.

On the 27th of November, 1876, I directed her to sit over hot water and allow the piles to protrude through the external sphincter; I then penetrated the pile with the needle of the hypodermic syringe and injected ten drops of a mixture of equal parts of carbolic acid and glycerine; the pile was then returned; the pain was not severe, and soon subsided without any medication; next day she was much better; the pile did not protrude the fifth day after the injection she was discharged cured. She then resumed her usual avocation. I ordered her a teaspoonful, three times daily, of the elixir of the phosphate of iron, quinine, and strychnia as a tonic, gentle out-door exercise and good nourishing food. After treatment she became pregnant—a primapara—and was confined without any return of the disease. Several years ago I treated her brother for the same disease, who informs me that he has had no return.

Lewis Everson, German, aged 45; laborer; was admitted into the Louisville City Hospital in July, 1877, with acute dysentery and intermittent fever. The latter part of August he was transferred to the surgical ward to be treated for frost-bite of the two great toes, which had been frosted two winters previous. The toes were removed by a member of the Surgical Staff 31st of August. When I took charge of the ward, September 1st, I found him weak, debilitated and feeble, still suffering from recurrent attacks of dysentery and intermittent fever, and hæmorrhoids which were much aggravated by the inflamed condition of the rectum and frequent straining at stool. By the 27th of September he had partially recovered from his complication of diseases, and was anxious to have something done for the piles, which came down when he walked or was at stool.

There were four large internal hæmorrhoids, which, when protruded formed a nodular circle around the mucous membrane of the rectum.

On the 29th of September, in presence of the medical class, I injected two of the hæmorrhoids with the following; Carbolic acid, drachms 1; aquæ distillat, drachms, 1; glycerin, drachms 1. M. S. Of which ten or twelve drops were injected into each of the piles. On the 1st of October I examined him, and found that the two injected piles had contracted and almost disappeared; I then injected the two remaining ones with the same injection, with equal quantity as before; by the 6th of October, Clinic day, he was again presented to the united classes and discharged. He suffered very little from the injection, and I was agreeably surprised at the rapid cure. He had two relapses of dysentery and malarial fever at intervals of about two and three weeks after the last injection, but no return of the piles. He was retained in the hospital until the latter part of November as assistant nurse in the ward, to give him time to recuperate his health, and to observe the result of the case. He had no further rectal trouble. His fever was controlled by sulphate of cinchonidia; after the paroxysms were interrupted he was ordered ferrum dialysatum twenty drops three times a day at meal time, sulphate cinchonidia five grains three times a day after eating, and special diet. While in the surgical ward the attacks of dysentery were treated as follows: R.—Bismuth subcarb., drachms ij; saccharat d pepsin, drachms 1½; morph., grs., ij. M F. Pulv. No. viij. S. one powder every two or four hours pro re nata; anodyne injections to control the straining; diet chiefly boiled sweet milk, with one table spoonful of wheat flour added to each pint. This case I consider an excellent test of the value and efficacy of the carbolic acid treatment in hæmorrhoids. Here is a man who had been prostrated with a complication of disease, enfeebled, anæmic, his sytem poisoned with malaria, who, for more than two years, had been suffering with ulcerated frosted toes, and laboring under all the inconveniences of an impecunious man.

The advantages of this treatment over the ligature are made manifest by comparison. August 31, the day before I took charge of the surgical ward, a patient about the same age had been ligatured for piles; the ligatures came away from the sixth to the tenth day, but he suffered much pain; the ulcers left after the separation of the ligatures healed slowly, and he did not recover for at least two or three weeks after the patient I operated on a month later was well and doing duty in the ward. For the injection of hæmorrhoids, carbolic acid has been combined with sweet oil or glycerine. At first I used carbolic acid and glycerine, equal parts, but I found this combination too thick to flow through the needle of the ordinary pocket hypodermic syringe. By having a needle made longer and larger in calibre it would answer the purpose very well. When I used equal parts of water and glycerine with the carbolic acid the solution flowed easily through the common hypodermic needle. Where the hæmorrhoids are recent and the walls of the veins not thickened, I used equal parts of carbolic acid, glycerine and distilled water, shake well for one or two minutes and you have a clear, uniform solution. Where the hæmorrhoids are of longer standing, the walls of the veins thickened and the connective tissue infiltrated with plastic material, the result of adhesive inflammation, I use two parts of the acid and one each of the glycerine and distilled water. Before operating, the patient's bowels should be evacuated by a mild laxative—magnesia or castor oil answers the purpose very well, aided, if necessay, by a warm water enema—then direct the patient to sit over a tub of warm water to relax the sphincters and protrude the piles; draw from ten to twenty drops of the acid solution, according to the size of the tumors, into the hypodermic syringe; pass the point of the needle through the most prominent part of the hæmorrhoid well into the cavity, then slowly inject the fluid, and hold it for a minute or two before withdrawing. A few drops of blood will flow from the puncture which is readily arrested by pressing over it a dossil of cotton wool; after the injection is completed return the pile within the sphincter and the operation is completed. The acid acts as an astringent, antiseptic and antiphlosgistic. No inflammation occurred in either of the cases referred to; but should it occur, use opiate suppositories, hot fomentations to the anus, keep the patient quiet and nourish with extract of beef and milk for a few days; give quinine and tr. ferri. mur. if indicated. After recovery the patient should be advised to avoid constipation, drastic purgatives, to use nourishing diet—meats, vegetables, cereals and fruits—a mixed diet, but not too great a variety at any one meal; it should be partly of a laxative character. If the bowels are sluggish, aid peristaltic action by drinking a teaspoonful of common table salt, in half a pint of warm water one hour before breakfast, or the same quantity of some of the laxative mineral waters; these are both prophylactic and curative; the "Tamar Indien" will act well where the patient can afford to buy them. An excellent, pleasant and palatable laxative in the treatment of piles or habitual constipation is the compound liquorice powder of the "Prussian Pharmacopœia;" viz.: R.—Fol. senna pulv., drachms ij; radix liquorice pulv., drachms ij; fœniculi sem. (German) pulv., drachms i; sulphurus depurati, drachms j; sacchar alb. pulv., drachms vi. M. S. a teaspoonful in a wine glass of water pro re nata.

There are many other laxatives which the peculiarities of each case will suggest. Rubbing the abdomen once or twice daily with salt water, and kneading thoroughly with the hands will often produce the desired result without any internal medication, provided the patient can be convinced of the efficacy of this kind of manual manipulation, and is not too indolent and indifferent to faithfully carry it out. System has much to do in relieving costipation; have a regular hour of the day to go to stool, lay aside all else, punctually attend to this duty, and the peristaltic action of the intestinal canal will keep time as accurately as the works of a twenty-four hour clock, provided the good house wife winds it up daily at the appointed hour. In case of general debility give some of the bitter tonics with iron in some form; plenty of sunlight, well ventilated apartments, suitable clothing and open air exercise. For patients of sedentary habits or indoor life prescribe a journey to the mountains, hunting, fishing, or a visit to some of the watering places, lay study and brain work and sedentary habits aside, seek cheerful society and recreation, forget the old infirmity and it will forget you. Patients are prone to neglect little things which, if looked to, will keep them well; they must be impressed with the fact that the body is like a piece of complex machinery, nicely adjusted and adapted in all its parts for its work, but to keep it so, it must be daily watched and cared for.

A few words in regard to the general treatment of piles. The special treatment of individual cases must be governed by the causes; these are local or temporary and constitutional or organic; of the former we have drastic purgatives, habitual constipation, dysentery, constant riding on horseback, standing, or sitting in a constrained posture, portal congestion, pregnancy, etc.; of the latter, organic disease of the stomach, liver, heart, or lungs, abdominal tumors which interfere with venous circulation. In the former a radical cure may be expected, in the latter only temporary relief, or if cured, other branches of the hæmorrhoidal veins will, from continuance of the cause, become dilated and reproduce the disease. Where the cause is local, and the veins not too much distended, general treatment with injections of hot or cold water, according to the feelings of the patients, is all that is necessary. Where the disease is of longer standing, and the veins much dilated, accompanied with general congestion, give such laxatives, tonics, and alteratives as each case suggests. Locally use enemas of water, or water and glycerine, or mucilage incorporated with persulphate of iron, or the vegetable astringents, adding in painful cases an anodyne of hyoscyamus, belladonna, stramonium or opium. If there is much tenderness and irritability, enemas of subnitrate or subcarbonate of bismuth, or carbolic acid in mucilage or glycerine and water will have a happy effect, to which an opiate may be added when indicated. The enemas should be small, not more than one or two ounces, if large the distension of the rectum will cause peristaltic action and discharge of the enema. Cotton-wool saturated with a solution of persulphate of iron has a good effect, especially in bleeding piles. The injection into the cavity of the dilated veins of a solution of the persulphate or perchloride of iron or ergot is dangerous, a portion of the coagulum formed may at any time be detached, carried into the circulation and produce embolism. Of late years I have generally used these various local remedies, alone or combined, in the form of suppositories by incorporating with cocoa butter, ten or fifteen grains to each suppository, and direct one to be used two or three times a day as required. If the patient can not readily introduce the suppository, order a suppository syringe, which can be passed into the anus, and deposit it at the proper place. I have never been partial to the nitric acid treatment; in the flat variety of hæmorrhoids with broad base, thickening of the mucous membrane and enlargement of the mucous papillæ, it might be used with advantage, but where the veins are much distended and the tumors well defined, I would not use it; the ligature is much to be preferred. In external piles, where they are pediculated with small base or like vegetations, clip them off with the scissors or scalpel; where they are tense with large base, soft and fluctuating, puncture and press out the blood; where they are hard and firm from thickening of the vein walls and blood clot, lay open with a bistory and press out the blood, then apply compresses; if tender and inflamed use hot fomentations and a T bandage If the walls of the veins and connective tissue have, from repeated inflammatory action, become consolidated and form hardened ridges or tumors, incise the skin and dissect out the hardened tissues, then close the wound and dress to get union by first intention. This treatment has been much more satisfactory than the local use of leaches for depletion and astringent unguents. This is very briefly an outline of my treatment for hæmorrhoids prior to the use of the carbolic acid injection. I have had no experience as yet in the treatment recommended by Mr. H. A. Reeves, of the London Hospital, which he calls "the immediate cure;" it consists in puncturing the pile to the base with a conical-pointed wire heated to a dull red heat; the number of punctures are governed by the size of the pile.

The common diseases of the rectum, viz., fistula, fissure, ulcer, and piles, the latter by far the most frequent, from some one of which few persons in a life-time escape, have from some unaccountable reason been considered the opprobria of surgery. Why should this be so? Why is it that the last two inches of the nether extremity of the alimentary canal, a plain piece of tubular anatomy, closed by two muscles, always ready to open at nature's call, supplied and nourished by the inferior hæmorrhoidal artery, and connecting veins, should be the prey of advertisers and specialists? The diseases are readily recognised by digital or specular examination, very amenable to treatment, much more easily cured than many other surgical cases, and are in themselves, neither dangerous nor fatal. Any surgeon of good common sense and judgment who is posted in his department, is as competent, yes, more competent, to treat this class of cases than the great mass of specialists who flood the country and cities with their fulsome circulars guaranteeing a certain cure, and certifying that no patient has ever died in their hands—*never died*—for the good reason that a patient about to die of some organic complication is always advised to go home and recuperate *for death;* the so-called doctor of secret remedies, known only to himself, has the fat fee in his pocket, the deluded and confident patient never returns, or if too feeble to leave, he is abandoned to his fate.

That there is wide spread prejudice against the surgeon's treatment of piles among the populace and even doctors, I am sorry to say, can not be denied. This is probably due; first, to the old-time treatment of excision by the knife and application of the actual cautery, to arrest the hæmorrhage, which has long since been abandoned. Second. The ethics of the Profession prevent the surgeon from advertising in the secular press and by circulars, giving certificates and names of prominent patients cured, which reach the populace. Third. The general practitioners, whose time is absorbed in the study and treatment of medical cases, do not advise their patients to consult the regular surgeons. Fourth. The advertising specialists are bold and confident, if they do learn what they know at the expense of the patient. They guarantee a cure without the use of the knife, ligature, or caustic, consulation free, and fifty, one hundred or two hudred dollars in advance, or negotiable notes. This means business; it is the charm; it fixes the patient; no knife, no ligature, no cautery, secret remedies, known only to the advertiser; the old Indian dodge—money in advance, never returned, cure or no cure. From these and other causes not necessary to mention, the mass of rectal diseases are treated outside of the regular Profession. The patients pay enormous fees, are satisfied in the belief that the regular surgeons know nothing of the remedies used, and that a mystery enshrouds the outlet of the rectum unknown to the ordinary mortals.

For two or three years past the injection of carbolic acid and oil or glycerine has been extensively used as a secret remedy. In portions of Illinois, Indiana, Tennessee, Kentucky, and other States, the right to use it in a prescribed territory has been sold for sums of money varying from five to fifteen hundred dollars, each purchaser being sworn to secrecy. Doctors, farmers, tradesmen, and sharpers, who could raise the "wherewith," have left their legitimate business and gone forth, armed with a hypodermic syringe and a bottle of carbolic acid and sweet oil to slay the rectal piles and gobble up a golden fortune. The discovery of valuable gold mines in the rectum is of comparatively recent date; the hypodermic syringe is more easily wielded than the pick and the shovel; no danger of Indians there and no scalps lost. Only a few days ago a prominent druggist informed me that an illiterate countryman, in Kentuck jeans, purchased his outfit and inquired if the oil would pass through the hypodermic needle. When asked what use he would make of the hypodermic syringe and acid oil mixture, he replied; "Gwine to practice medicine; right smart sprinkling of piles whar I live." A sad case of this territorial selling deception came under my own observation: A few months ago an intelligent looking gentleman, in delicate health, a stranger to me, called at my office and enquired for a certain number of Braithwait's Retrospect,

stating that he wished to see an article on the use of cabolic acid and
sweet oil in the treatment of piles. I stated that I had not read the article referred to, but I had seen the treatment briefly mentioned in other
journals, and that I had, for more than a year, been using the acid and
glycerine, He then stated he was a regular physician, had practiced in
Kentucky for several years, had been unable to attend to general practice,
his means were well nigh exhausted, had a family to support. In looking around to find some way to make a support, he heard of this secret
remedy for the treatment of piles. He consulted some of his friends
about the propriety of giving fifteen hundred dollars for the secret remedy and a specified territory to operate in. Among these friends was a
prominent practitioner of this city, who advised the invalid doctor to make
the purchase. The purchase was made, the contract drawn, the papers
duly signed, the secret imparted, the territory assigned, and when the vic-,
timised doctor reached the field of operation, he learned, to his astonish-
ment, that the secret was public property. The object of his inquiry of
me was to get sufficient evidence against the party in this city who had
sold the alleged secret remedy, to institute suit for obtaining money under
false pretenses, and compel the return of the money. Now if a regular
practitioner, whose locks have been silvered in the service, who claims to
observe the proprieties of the profession, who is tenacious for its honor,
will volunteer such advice, will encourage such quackery, what can the
profession hope for? If men of influence sanction advertisers and secret
nostrums, what becomes of medical ethics? This man is a teacher of
medicine; what an ignoble example to place before the rising generation
of doctors. O temporal O mores!!— *The American Medical Bi-Weekly.* '-

An Epidemic Traced.

Dr. Russell has just published a brilliant report on the epidemic of enteric fever, which has been prevalent in the west end of Glasgow and the
west end suburbs of Hillhead. He traces the steps by which he pursued
the inquiry into the sources of the infection, and no one can read his report without being convinced that here again we have an epidemic trace-
able to infection through milk. We shall tell the tale, not as Dr. Russell
does, but rather in the order of time, and with all possible brevity. In a
picturesque situation, on the banks of the Avon, stands a farm, whose ar-
rangements are such as to favor the contamination of the products of the
dairy. In this farm a son sickened with enteric fever on December 1,
a servant girl on December 20, and another boy on December 27. The

work of the dairy was carried on by persons who attended the patients. From this farm there were sent daily twenty-five gallons of milk to Messrs. Semple & Wilson, of Hillhead, and they passed on eight gallons to Messrs. Morrisons. The seventeen gallons retained were distributed to families in Hillhead and the west end of Glasgow, partly to wholesale and retail customers. The immediate result was an epidemic of enteric fever, almost entirely among the customers of Messrs. Semple & Wilson and Messrs. Morrisons. The manner in which the disease picked out the persons using infected milk is most graphically shown, by one or two examples appended by Dr. Russell, which we may quote.

"In Hill Street, (Garnethill) there are seven families supplied with suspected milk, of whom three are infected, and a hundred and eighty-one supplied otherwise, not one of whom is infected. In Berkeley Terrace there is one family supplied with suspected milk, which is infected, and thirty-seven otherwise supplied, not one of whom is infected. In Royal Terrace there is only one family supplied with suspected milk, which is infected, and twenty eight which is otherwise supplied, not one of whom is infected. In Lynedoch Crescent there are two families supplied with suspected milk, of whom one is infected and fifteen otherwise supplied, not one of whom is infected. In Park Street East, there are five families supplied with suspected milk, of whom one is infected, and twelve otherwise supplied, not one of whom is infected. In Park Circus there are nine families supplied with suspected milk, of whom two are infected, and twenty-seven otherwise supplied, not one of whom is infected. In Woodlands Terrace there are seven families supplied with suspected milk, of whom five are infected, and fourteen supplied otherwise, not one of whom is in fected. In Park Gardens two families are supplied with suspected milk one of whom is infected, and four supplied otherwise, not one of whom is infected. In Clairmount Terrace there are seven families supplied with suspected milk, of whom three are infected, and five supplied otherwise, not one of whom is infected. In Woodside Crescent there are four families supplied with suspected milk, one of whom is infected, and thirteen supplied otherwise, not one of whom is infected. Another area of infection is amongst the students of the University, who, on the 21st of December, were dispersed over the country for their Christmas Holidays. There are now some absentees from illness and I have obtained the names of seven of these who have already been discovered to have enteric fever. Of that small number three are now dead—at Kilwinning, at Langloan, and in Islay The refreshment room in the University was supplied with milk by Semple & Wilson. It was largely patronized by the students, and those men are known to have partaken of the milk."

Dr. Russell may well remark that, in this epidemic, we have as clear an experiment performed for us as in any of the demonstrations of the chemists' laboratory.—*From The British Medical Journal.*

BY
J. MILNER FOTHERGILL, M. D.
M. R. C. P. Lond.

The title of this paper is brief, and perhaps a more accurate but long and clumsy title would be "A Form of Dyspepsia induced and kept up by Irritation arising from the Ovary," *i. e.*, disturbance in the stomach may be excited reflexly by irritation situated in another viscus. No attempt will be made here to enter into the literature of ovarian disorders. It is enough to say that the various maladies of the ovary, other than gross organic changes, as cystic tumors, have not received the attention they merit. Barnes has referred to them in his recent work on the Diseases of Women (quoting Charcot and Negrier), and Lombe Atthill has worked at them. The attention of the writer was drawn to the subject in a round-a-bout rather than a direct way.

It will perhaps place the subject most clearly before the reader to relate briefly how it came about. It was observed that a large number of the patients attending the City of London Hospital for Diseases of the chest, with consolidation of one or other apex, night sweats, or heightened temperature, loss of flesh, and the other symptoms of phthisis, had a good family history. The patient too often had a good physique and the lung mischief might fairly be set down to accidental causes rather than a family predisposition to phthisis. This was a very unsatisfactory state of matters, and it was evidently desirable to investigate the cases further. The two main concomitants of these cases of phthisis were soon seen to be dyspepsia, with leucorrhoea and menorrhagia—a combined condition common with women. Here there were linked a defective body in comon with an excessive body expenditure, producing a condition of general malnutrition, just the condition favorable to the development of tubercle. For some time it was thought that this association of dispepsia and disturbance in the sexual organs was a mere casual one. It appeared that the leucorrhea had existed some time with or without mennorrhagia, and then that the stomach became disturbed, and a dyspeptic condition established. But a little further attention to the subject soon showed that the connection was much more decided than this. It was seen that the condition was not merely one where the system had for some time been taxed by heavy body-expenditure, against which it had kept up as long as the nutritive processes were efficiently carried on; and then that from some cause, psychial or physical, disturbance of the digestion was set up, and then the nutrition distinctly failed With an impaired nutrition the system could no longer withstand the excessive expenditure, and then tubercle followed. This explanation was sufficient as regards the genesis of tubercle, but was insufficient and unsatisfactory in other respects. The connection of gastric disturbance with irritation in the genito-urinary system stood in a very suggestive relationship to this complex condition. It is well known that vomiting is a constant symptom of a calculus in the pelvis of the kidney. The vomiting of early months of pregnancy when the embryonic muscular fibres of the uterus are commencing to develop and take on a more active condition, has been long a notorious fact. It soon became clear that there was some condition existing which stood in a causal relationship to both the dyspepsia and uterine disturbance. That condition was quickly seen to be a state of vascular excitement in one or both ovaries, usually the left ovary. This condition Barnes terms oophoria.

In this state there is always more or less pain constantly in the iliac fossa, more rarely on the right, much aggravated at the catamenial periods, when the pain shoots from the turgid ovary down the thigh of the coresponding side along the genito-crural nerve. This painful state is otherwise known as "ovarian dysmenorrhea." When pressure is made over this tender ovary during the catamenial flow, acute pain is experienced. Pressure also elicits pain during the intermenstrual interval. At the same time that acute pain is felt, evidence is furnished of emotional perturbation, the patient feels as if about to faint, "or feels queer all over," as some express it, and the changes in the patient's countenance speak of something more than mere pain, pure and simple. It is evident there is a wave of nerve-perturbation set up, which excites more than to sensation of pain. Commonly the patient feels sick after the momentary pressure, and asks to be permitted to sit down, alleging that she feels sick and faint. If careful physical examination be made it will be found that there is an enlarged and tender ovary, which may sometimes be caught betwixt the finger in the vagina and the finger of the other hand applied to the abdominal wall over the ovary. Such manipulation elicits manifestations of acute suffering from the patient. Frequently the rectus muscle over the tender ovary is hard and rigid, so as to place the organ as perfectly at rest as possible; just as we see the rectus to stiffen and become rigid over the liver when there is an hepatic abscess and thus to secure rest, as regards movement, for that viscus.

We have then a morbid condition of a very important, if small organ, and can comprehend how this can set up waves of nerve-perturbation which will be felt in distant organs. The disturbances so excited are not the same in all cases. The waves so set up may break on several points. In one the stomach is perturbed, in another palpitation is induced, in a third a neurosal cough is excited; in almost all there is neuralgia of the sixth or seventh intercostal nerve, I believe always, or very frequently, to be quite safe, on the same side as the affected ovary. Certainly left side intercostal neuralgia is much commoner than right side neuralgia of the intercostal nerves; as much commoner as left oophoria is than 'right oophoria. It appeared that the nerve-currents set up in the ovary travelled along the dorsal ganglia till the splanchnics were reached, and then their force was most felt in the intercostal nerves at the point where the greater splanchnics run off. When talking the subject over one day with Dr. Mitchell Bruce, he reminded me that the nerve fibres of the splanchnics were descending fibres chiefly. My hypothesis is this: the currents ascending from the ovary, of which some reach the brain as sentient pain, possibly along the sympathetic, are met by the descending currents passing into the greater splanchnics, and driven off thereby on to the neigboring intercostal nerves, the sixth or seventh. The perturbations set up in the ovary are thus felt in the terminal fibres of these intercostal nerves as gusts of neuralgic pain.

At the same time there is uterine disturbance excited. Usually the womb is heavy and turgid, and the os patulous or uneven and harder than usual. There is commonly menorrhagia; there is always leucorrhœa. Less frequently there is a condition of imperfect or lessened menstrual hemorrhage, with a persistent and profuse leucorrhœa. Not rarely, too, there is set up a very distressing condition, viz., that of recurring orgasm. This occurs most commonly during sleep, "the period par excellence of reflex excitability." In more aggravated cases it also occurs during the waking moments; and this it does without any reference to psychical conditions. It is found alike in the married woman cohabiting with her husband, and in spinsters who might be suspected of regretting their involuntary continence. It is not certainly due to repression of the sexual instinct. My experience is clear about that. Woman is much calumniated as to the origin of many of her troubles. When this condition of recurrent orgasm is established, it at times leads to a still more distressing condition, viz., a state at once of weakness and irritability of the bladder centres in the lumbar portion of the spinal cord. The centres or the pelvic viscera lie near together in the cord, and the condition of one is readily communicated to another. The brief recurrent orgasm affects the bladder centres, and the call to make water is sudden and imperative, and must be attended to at once, or a certain penalty be paid for non-attention. This last is not a common condition, fortunately, but it is a source of great suffering, mental and bodily, when it does occur. The condition of the ovary also acts reflexly upon the uterus, and keeps it in a state of persistent erection and high vascularity, with the normal phenomena attendant thereupon. This enables us readily to comprehend the uterine associations of this complex malady, both as regards the leucorrhœa and the menorrhagia. That sometimes, instead of menorrhagia there is a condition rather of intensified leucorrhœa than a true menstrual flux, is what we can readily understand. The rythmic wave of supplemental nutrition, which reaches its climax in the menstrual hemorrhage, is sorely interfered with, and instead of an escape of blood, there is a flow of fluid scarcely tinged with blood. The starved organism is no longer equal to the period-ic hemorrhage. Nevertheless the accumulated discharge during each month is far beyond the sum total of the generative expenditure of a per-fectly healthy woman. So much for the uterine half of the complex condition.

Now for the gastric side of the question. The stomach contains sym-pathetic nerve-fibres, isolated nerve-ganglia, with some fibres of the pneu-mogastric. These last fibres have an antagonistic or inhibatory influence over the sympathetic fibres of the stomach; the sympathetic fibres pro-duce contraction of the blood-vessels, the pneumogastric fibres tend to produce dilatation. Thus Claude Bernard found that section of the gas-tric branches of the vagus stopped digestion, and the mucous membrane of the stomach, previously turgid with blood, became pale and ceased to secrete. Further, "the influence of the pneumogastric nerves over the secretion of gastric fluid has been of late even more decidedly shown by M. Bernard, who found that galvanic stimulus of these excited nerves exci-ted an active secretion of fluid; while a like stimulus applied to the sym-pathetic nerves issuing from the semilunar ganglia, caused a diminution and even complete arrest of the secretion." This quotation is not from any recent work on physiology, but from an old edition of the text-book of the late Senhouse Kirkes. These experiments of M. Bernard have been performed by others with like results. Thus we see that the effects of a stimulus, applied to the sympathetic nerves of the stomach, cause a dimi-nution and even complete arrest of the gastric secretion. Is there any dif-ficulty then in comprehending the relations betwixt dyspepsia, and an ir-ritable condition of an organ with which the stomach is in intimate con-nection through its sympathetic fibres? The relations of dyspepsia to a disturbed ovary become clear enough. The irritation set up in the ovary traverses the sympathetic fibres and arrests the flow of gastric juice, more or less thoroughly, and dyspepsia is the consequence. The action of the sympathetic nerve-fibrils is to excite contraction of the arteries and arte-rioles; that of the pneumogastric fibrils to dilate them.

Persistent nerve-currents coming up, the sympathetic nerve fibrils ex-cite them, and contraction of the blood-vessels is the result. The termi-nation of the nerve-currents starting from the ovary is the contraction of the gastric blood-vessels. Just as we know that perturbations set up by a calculus in the kidney, or the growing uterus, will flow on until they reach the stomach and cease in the act of vomiting. The dyspepsia is then the direct and immediate consequence of the ovarian irritation. The disturbance of the stomach is due to far-away irritation—it is not prima-ry, but reflex.

This condition of contraction of the gastric blood-vessels, with arrest of gastric secretion, leads to dyspepsia, and the imperfect digestion of the food taken. In the act of digestion the blood vessels of the stomach dilate, the mucous membrane becomes turgid with blood, and the secretion of gastric juice is abundant. These waves coming up, the sympathetic fibres disturb these processes, the dilatation of the blood-vesels is interfered with, the secretion of gastric juice checked, and impaired digestion follows. Thus we can see distinctly enough the gastric factor of this complex condition.

The dyspepsia and the uterine flux are alike the consequences of a condition standing to each in a causal relationship. The imperfect body income and the increased body expenditure alike arise from and are excited by a certain condition of the ovary.

How the ovary becomes affected in the first instance it is not easy to say. Following the suggestions of John Williams that in these cases there had always existed a certain amount of pain at menstruation from its first initiation, a series of inquiries were instituted. In a certain proportion of instances such seemed to have been the case. But in the bulk of cases there was no such history, and the disturbance dated from a definite point. In many this was a miscarriage, in others an acute illness, in a few marriage, and in middle-aged women getting near the end of their reproductive life, commonly a confinement. In young women in their 'teens it seemed due to an excess of the usual ovarian excitement set up by the changes of puberty; in not a few from the effects of working treadle sewing-machines, the evil effects of which on some girls are now notorious. The most difficult part of the entire subject is the etiology.

Once this condition of the ovary established, then a whole train of disturbances follow in its wake. In some cases there is a neurosal cough, a pharyngeal cough, identical in its reflex nature with the cough of pregnancy, known in Scotland as "a cradle cough." In others there is palpitation, as reflex in its nature as the palpitation induced by a prolapsed uterus, and which is relieved as soon as the uterus is replaced in its normal position. The wave of nerve-perturbation set up in the ovary passes onward till it reaches a terminus where its vibrations excite local disturbance. When the brunt of this wave falls upon the stomach it produces contraction of the gastric arterioles with defective secretion of gastric juice; the digestive act is imperfect, and imperfect assimilation and nutrition follows. These perturbations, too, affect the normal contractions of the stomach in the digestive act, and instead of the ordinary movements of digestion, such contractions as produce vomiting are excited. Such is the true pathology of those cases of obstinate vomiting, or rejection of food, as it is often termed, seen in girls of from nineteen to three or four and twenty years of age, with which all experienced practitioners are familiar. The medical attendant is nearly worried out of his life; the friends of the patient are worked up to a feverish anxiety; the sufferings of the patient herself are not inconsiderable; and so the case wears on for weeks. The vomiting persists; the moment any food is taken into the stomach and the digestive act commences, the food is rejected, and, in dispair, feeding by the rectum has to be adopted. As remedies, bismuth, opium, hydrocyanic acid, effervescing mixtures, champagne, milk and soda-water, beef-tea, hot and cold, raw meat pounded, all are tried and fail—are abandoned in dispair, and nutritive enemata are the last resort. All who have seen much practice are familiar with these trying cases, which seem to go on unaffected by remedial measures, until the malady seems to wear itself out; to be succeeded by a long and tedious convalescence. It would seem that at least the condition of general mal-nutrition starves down the congested ovary till it ceases to set up and send out those perturbative nerve-currents which excite the gastric disturbance. Then the stomach settles down and resumes its ordinary duties once more without disorder. The case lingers on unrelieved because its real pathology is not recognized. The stomach is treated, and not the ovary. The gastric disturbance is not primary, but reflex. Its causation must be comprehended, and the treatment directed accordingly, and then improvement will follow.

An illustrative case may be mentioned. It is not so well marked as the aggravated case just given in the above sketch; for these cases are only met with in private practice in their most developed form. A girl of twenty-two was sent into the West London Hospital as a case of long-continued retching and vomiting. The house surgeon gave her an effervescing mixture containing hydrocyanic acid, which gave some relief. The girl was pale and anæmic, with lack-lustre eyes, and a peculiar expression about her which made me at once feel sure that she was the subject of ovarian disturbance. It was found at once that the left ovary was congested and exqusitely tender, pressure over it almost leading to syncope. There were also menorrhagia and leucorrhœa. The ovary was treated, and in ten days the girl left the hospital well; but I doubt if permanently cured. And yet this stomach had been treated nobody knows how long wihout avail.

What is the treatment of these cases? It consists of several factors, each essential and complementary to the other. In the first place the bowels must be thoroughly opened. Any load in them will always increase pelvic congestion. They must be well opened every morning and also emptied at bed time. It is very bad for these cases to have any load in the lower bowel during sleep. The best purgative is sulphate of magnesia. It may be given alone or with aloes. Aloes in small doses excites the hemorrhoidal vessels, in full doses relieves them. Mineral waters containing sulphate of magnesia may be used. Free purgation should be first set up, and then an open condition of the bowels maintained. If the stomach rejects all medicines, they must be given in enemata. But by means of a hypodermic injection of morphia in a full dose, the stomach can usually be soothed into tolerating medicines. If necessary, a morphia suppository at bedtime may be ordered. Purgation acts directly upon the ovary and lowers its excitability.

Then comes the treatment of the reflexly excited disorder. It is obvious that such remedies as bismuth and hydrocyanic acid act locally upon the stomach, and so, though no doubt of value, are after all but palliative measures. Instead of treating the stomach it is necessary to act upon the nerve-tracts, along which the perturbing nerve-currents travel. For this purpose the great therapeutic agent is bromide of potassium. It affects (as pointed out at length in the Practitioner's Handbook of Treatment) alike the peripheral ends of the nerves and nerve-fibres; it blunts the nerve-endings; it lessens nerve conductivity while it lowers central receptivity.

By its use in full doses the excitement in the ovary and the perturbative waves set up thereby are diminished; and the path obstructed so that by the time the wave has reached the stomach it is greatly reduced in force; and perhaps never reaches the stomach at all, but gets lost on the way. The formula in ordinary use is as follows:

Magnesia Sulphas,................................drachms i.
Potassa Bromidum,.................................scruples i.
Inf. Gentian,......................................ounces i.

three times a day; with an aloes and myrrh pill at bedtime, if necessary. The gentian acts beneficially on the stomach, as all bitters do. and renders it more tolerant of the medicines. A vehicle for the chief remedial agents need not be taken haphazard, but selected.

Counter-irritation is very useful. A blister may be placed over the tender ovary. It should be put on as the first step. It certainly affects the patient's mind favorably, and it does positive good physically. It usually produces such an impression that the medicines given by the mouth are tolerated by the stomach. As to how such counter-irritation acts we do not yet quite know. But we are well assured that it does act and efficiently too. Probably one nerve-wave may meet and neutralize another, like rays of light. Ferrier (The Functions of the Brain) writes, "Though, as a rule, the summation of stimuli increases the reflex action and makes it more general, this is only true of stimuli conveyed to the same part of the cord (Wundt). If, on the other hand, a sensory nerve in some other part of the body is simultaneously irritated, then the reflex action which would otherwise result from the first stimulus is altogether restrained or inhibited (Herzen, Schiff)." The impressions or nerve-currents excited by a blister over the ovary and outside the abdominal walls, would necessarily travel some distance before they meet those set up within the ovary. An ordinary fly blister, two inches square, suits very well. It perhaps produces the best effects when placed right over the tender ovary. In two instances a crop of boils followed the blister. But this is less than one per cent, of all the cases.

By such means the disease must be treated. There remain the increased body expeniture and the imperfect body income still to be considered.

For the first—the vaginal loss—injections of astringents in solution by means of a Higginson's syringe, or the small india rubber ball and tube used to give babies enemata (much better in every way than a glass syringe) must be used twice a day, with hip baths daily, if the patient's condition will admit of it. This is far from unimportant. When there is menorrhagia, quietude and the ovoidance of all warm drinks and food during the flow are desirable. For the latter—the imperfect digestion—light and easily digestible food, milk, if necessary, combined with an alkali, or beef-tea with a little cream in it, or custard, are indicated. Such food should be given at short intervals, and small quantities at once. The irritable stomach will often retain small quantities of food when larger amounts are at once rejected. But after all this last is but palliative treatment of these cases they are not primary stomach affections, they are truly reflex, and the origin of the malady must be ascertained, after which comes the appropriate and essential treatment. So frequently does dyspepsia in women depend causally upon ovarian mischief, that the writer now always commences by eliminating the ovarian factor before treating the malady as a pure stomach affection.—*From American Journal of Obstetrics.*

A BILL.

For an Act Entitled an Act to Regulate the Practice of Medicine, Surgery and Obstetrics; and also to Regulate the Vending of Drugs, and to Punish Offenders for the Violation of the same.

SEC. 1. *Be it Enacted by the General Assembly of the State of Iowa,* On and after the 4th day of July, A. D., 1878, it will be unlawful for any person to engage in the practice of medicine and surgery, or for any druggist or drug clerk to dispense or combine by prescription, or otherwise, any drug or medicine without first obtaining his or her certificate of qualification as in this act made and provided.

SEC. 2. Any person desiring to engage in the practice of medicine, surgery and obstetrics, within the meaning of this act, shall make application to the county auditor for an order to appear before the Iowa state board of health for his or her examination. Upon the payment into the treasury of the county in which the applicants propose to practice, the fees, all necessary charges as hereinafter provided, the county auditor will issue said order. If the candidate for said certificate of qualification be a legal holder of a diploma, issued from any regularly chartered medical school or university of America or Europe, will be entitled to a certificate of his or her qualification, upon presenting the receipt of the county treasurer of amount of $1.00 fees paid, together with his or her diploma, and evidence that the person named in said diploma is the holder thereof; that it was legally issued from a reputable school of medicine and surgery, and not from a school or university noted for dealing in "bogus" diplomas, and also such further evidence as said state board of health may require to fully satisfy them that the candidate for certificate of qualification actually made the studies as set forth in the diploma; in which case, upon recording his or her legitimate diploma, together with his or her certificate of qualification aforesaid, and the payment of the usual charges for recording the same in the recorder's office in the county in which said physician proposes to practice the profession within the meaning of this act, and upon full compliance with all the provisions of this act, said person will be entitled to all its privileges and benefits.

SEC. 3. Any person not a graduate in medicine and surgery, who has been engaged in the reputable practice of medicine and Surgery, for a period of ten years within the limits of this state, may make application to the county auditor of the county in which he or she proposes to practice, and by the payment of a fee of ($26,00) twenty six dollars into the county treasury and all necessary. charges for recording, as in preceding section, the applicant will be entitled to a receipt for the amount so paid, and also to an order to appear before said Iowa state board of health to submit to his or her exmination as to qualification to practice medicine, surgery and obstetrics within the meaning of this act; and upon the receipt of said certificate of qualification (which shall be valid for the period of two years from the date thereof,) and recording the same as provided in section 2 of this act, he or she will be entitled to all the rights and privileges of this act.

SEC. 4. Any person appearing before said Iowa state board of health for a certificate of qualifications, based on the merits of fraudulently obtained, forged or bogus diploma, knowing the same to be such, or who seeks to obtain said certificate upon a legitimate diploma issued to a person other than to him or herself. or otherwise obtain or seeks to obtain such certificate fraudulently, upon an information filed by the order of said board of health, and upon conviction, will be punished by receiving the severest penalties for violations of this act,

SEC. 5. All persons obtaining certificates of qualifications based on ten years experience in practice of medicine and surgery, will be required, within two years from date of certificate, to finish their studies, by attending one or more full courses of instruction at any reputable medical school or university of America or Europe, and obtain a diploma, or be forever prohibited from practicing medicine, surgery and obstetrics, within the meaning of this act.

SEC. 6. Medical students of three years close study may practice the profession of medicine and surgery within the meaning of this act in connection with and under the direct supervison of a practicing physician, who has complied with all the provisions of this act; *provided,* said practicing physician legally assume all risk of damage done that may attach to said student by reason of his ignorance.

SEC. 7. Nothing in this act will prohibit any intelligent person from lending humane assistance in any case of accident or emergency when called upon; *provided,* the person so assisting will (in case the accident or emergency be one requiring skilled medical or surgical attendance) send or cause to be sent for immediately a physician and surgeon who has complied with the provisions of this act; *and provided further,* that said humane person make no claim or charge for said services.

SEC. 8. Any person taveling within the limits of this state as an itinerant physician or surgeon will be required to strictly conform to all the provisions of this act, and in addition thereto must pay one hundred dollars per month as a license (for the benefit of the temporary school fund) into the county treasury of the county in which said advertised itinerant physician or surgeon proposes to practice the profession, within the meaning of this act. Failing to comply with the provisions of this section. the offender will, upon conviction, receive the highest penalty of fine and imprisonment, as set forth in section No. 18 of this act.

SEC. 9. All physicians, surgeons and obstetricians practicing within the meaning of this act, upon receipt of the necessary blanks, with instruction, shall make and forward to the Iowa state board of health such quarterly or other reports as said board may ask of each member of the profession, as defined by section No. 17 of this act, and they shall keep such a journal of important cases in practice, and such register of observation, in manner and form. as said Iowa state board of health may direct. Failing to comply with this section subjects a penalty of ten dollars for each offense, collection enforced as other penalties, and paid into the county treasury for the benefit of the temporary school fund.

SEC. 10. Any physician, surgeon, obstetrician, druggist, or drug clerk, who, engaging in any practice, manipulation or procedure for the production of criminal abortion, by the use of instruments, appliances, drugs, nostrums or otherwise, knowing the same to be handled or administered for the express purpose of producing a miscarriage of any pregnant female, unless such miscarriage be necessary to save her life; or if any physician, surgeon, obtetrician, druggist or drug clerk advise with, suggest, educate or instruct irresponsible persons in means and procedure for producing criminal abortion; or in any manner whatever aid, encourage, countenance, or sanction, or in any manner be a party with intent to procure criminal abortion, by the sale, delivery, or instructing the party as to what means may be used successfully for the procurement of criminal abortion, upon conviction, shall be subject to existing penalties of chapter 2, section 3863. of Code of Iowa; and in addition thereto, his or her certificate of qualification shall be canceled by the court by entering on the judgment docket as part of findings of sentence, that the party so convicted has forfeited the rights and benefits of this act, unless the disability be specially removed by executive clemency.

SEC. 11. That it shall be unlawful for any druggist, apothecary, or drug clerk who are not graduates of legally incorporated colleges of pharmacy, either of America or Europe, to dispense drugs and medicine, or combine medicine by prescription, or otherwise, or handle drugs as a vender, without first obtaining a certificate of his or her qualification from a college of pharmacy, or from a board of examining commissioners, consisting of three members, of practical druggists, graduates from a legally incorporated college of pharmacy, who have been recommended to the governor of this state for his appointment by the pharmaceutical society of Iowa. In case there be no organized pharmaceutical society in this state, then the Iowa state board of health may recommend said commissioners to the governor for his appointment. Said commissioners, when qualified, shall examine all applicants who present themselves for examination with an order for examination from the county auditor, and a receipt from the county treasurer that he or she has paid the sum of twenty-six dollars as a fee, which shall be for the benefit of the temporary board of health fund, of the county in which the party propose to vend drugs. Said examining commissioners shall certify the result of their examination to the Iowa state board of health, who will issue their certificate of qualification, and upon recording his or her certificate of qualification, as made and provided in section 2 of this act, the person will be entitled to all the rights and privileges of this act.

SEC. 12. Each member of the examining commissioners, as provided for in section 11 of this act, will receive for each person examined, upon an order from county auditor, five dollars, to be paid out of the temporary Iowa board of health fund as hereinafter proveded.

SEC. 13. From and after the passage of this act, no medical student will be permitted to practice medicine within the meaning of this act without first obtaining a diploma from a legally chartered medical school, either of America or Europe, except as provided in section No. 6 of this act.

SEC. 14. From and after the passage of this act, no drug apprentice or clerk will be permitted to dispense drugs or medicine, by prescription or otherwise, within the limits of this state, without first obtaining a diploma from a college of pharmacy, either of America or Europe, except as provided in section No. 15 of this act.

SEC. 15. Nothing in this act will be construed to prohibit students, or apprentices of pharmacy, to handle drugs or medicines, provided the\ are under the direct supervision of practical druggists who have complied with all the requirements of this act, and who legally assume all responsibility which may attach to said apprentices' ignorance.

SEC. 16. For defraying the expenses incurred by reason of the act creating the Iowa state board of health, and also the act to regulate the practice of medicine, surgery, &c, it is hereby made and provided that the fees paid into the conty treasury, as provided in sections Nos. 2 3 and 11 of the act entitled "An to regulate the practice of medicine and surgery," &c., shall be known as the temporary board of health fund, and shall be paid into the state treasury quarterly, and shall be paid out upon warrants, as other funds are, and only for defraying expenses made by reason of this act.

SEC. 17. Physicians, surgeons and obstetricians will be only construed to mean persons who have satisfied the Iowa state board of health of their qualification and fitness to practice the various branches of the profession of medicine, surgery and obstetrics generally, or either branch specially. The evidence of qualification must be of record in the recorder's office, as provided in preceding section; otherwise they are not physicans, surgeons and obsterician within the meaning of this act.

Sec. 18. Any physician, surgeon, or obstetrician, druggist, apothecary, or drug clerk, who violates any of the provisions of this act, which may pertain to them, upon conviction, for the first offense, will be fined fifty dollars and the costs of the suit; for the second offense they will, upon conviction, be fined five hundred dollars, and imprisonment for one year, with costs of suit, and for each succeeding offense will be subject to like penalties.

SEC. 19, No physician, surgeon, obstetrician, druggist, or drug clerk, who are continuing in business in violation of this act shall obtain legal process for the collection of any claim or demand made or contracted in violation of this act.

House File No. 47.   Seaman.

We publish the above, a copy of the bill, House File No. 47 introduced in the house by Hon. Bruce Seaman, of Scott County. From the number of bills introduced, we select house file No. 47, as being perfect in every detail, and which will meet the wants of the profession, and protect the people from empiricism.

We have had years of personal acquaintance with Mr. Seaman, and feel assured that in him the bill will have an able advocate when it shall be put upon its passage.

The profession, and the people should lend every aid needed to Mr Seaman in his effort to raise the standard of qualification of the medical profession, in consequence of which, the people will be specially benefitted in preservation of health, and prolongation of life. ED.

NEWS.

The Present Number of the Journal---The Medical Law.

The influx of communications has been so copious of late, that, notwithstanding the almost complete surrender of the present issue to them, we have been compelled to postpone several important papers for the March number, and also to exclude the proceedings of the Sanfrancisco Microscopical Society. During the many years of our connection with medical journalism in California, there has been nothing to approach the present activity of the professional mind in the State, in the direction of literary development. We attribute this, with other good results, to the Medical Law, and the consequent action of the Board of Examiners, by which the entire profession, from one extremity of the State to the other, has been stirred up and vitalized. A few of the brethren who fixed their attention at the onset upon the defects of the law, have never yet been able to see anything but its defects. We would advise them to turn it over and look at the other side; and then, even if they cannot perceive good enough in it to counterbalance the evil, to fall into line with the great body of the profession in an effort to amend and improve it. Having gone thus far, with much cost and labor, it is prudent and discreet to adopt this course. *—From the Pacific Medical and Surgical Journal.*

QUACKERY.—In the last issue of this Journal the thanks of the Medical Profession were tendered the "Kentuckey Advocate" and the Weekly Local" (both published at Danville, Ky.,) for their successful efforts in suppressing the quackery of a peripatetic imposter who had been doing an injury to the Public in the Southern portion of this State. The "Weekly Local" claims that the "Advocate" is not entitled to any thanks; and constructively that it is entitled to all. Well! the "Advocate" is so uniformly entitled to the thanks of the Profession for its course that it can safely occupy the position accorded it.— *The American Medical Bi-Weekly.*

The secular press in this State occupy another position than be found clamoring for the honors of strangling the animal whose only qualifications are their brazen-faced impudence in assuming to be doctors of medicine, and their ability to secure the services of the artful news paper press to charm the victim, whilst he is being robbed of his health and means. There are no doubt many worthy exceptions, prominently among which we mention the Osceola *New Era*, as having contained a number of original articles, ably written, and in favor of the proposed legislation regulating the practice of Medicine and Surgery in this state, for which, we tender the thanks of the profession, and urge them to recognize the services.

Editorial.

We present the first number of the _Catlin_ to the Medical Profession of
Iowa, believing that it will supply the wants of many. In undertaking to
publish a Journal which will reflect credibly on the Editor: The State and
its worthy members of the profession, our entire physical and mental ener-
gies will be fully enlisted in the work, knowing that merit will surely receive the reward for patient, persistant toil.

It is not expected that our first feeble effort at Medical Journalism will
eclipse, or supplant any of the many signals of warning, which, for years
have guided the profession safely into harbor; but on the contrary, feeling our weakness, and only claiming the _Catlin_ to be a legitimate child of
the Profession, though erring, the kind parent will be solicitous for our
welfare, and will lend that approving smile for merit, without which, we
must go down in our own secretion.

The harbor for which the _Catlin_ has cleared, is "A higher Standard" of
attainments in the medical profession, to arrive at which, we will be compelled to measure shafts with advocates and defenders of charlatanism
near at hand, who will ever find the _Catlin_ keenly whetted (in justice to
the afflicted) to cut from this commonwealth, the foul infectious carcass of
professional ignorance. For the profession of medicine and surgery as it
is now practiced in the state of Iowa without legally prescribed qualifications, or attainments in professional education necessary that each member thereof should possess before assuming such an important trust, seriously endangers the lives of the people, and also unnecessarily swells the
mortuary reports.

The gross ignorance of many persons, who without necessary study or
preparation, and whose only qualifications are to assume to be doctors, and
pretend to practice Medicine: Their ignorance is so apparrant to the
averaged intellect, that this profession once called a science, for the want
of protective legislation, has degenerated into a curse, whose poisonous
shafts pierce the former objects of its mercies; In consequence of which,
the many worthy members of the profession, living within the state are
jealous of their science, and solicitous for its advancement, and for the
welfare of the people. They who have spent their entire lives in study
and toil for advancement in science, and relief from suffering, enter with
sickning disgust upon the task of strangling professional ignorance of eve-
ly theory or phase, by urging the present Legislature, to enact laws pre-

servative of the lives of the people by prescribing the qualification of physicians.

The evil complained of has greatly increased since a number of our neighboring states have enacted laws preservative of the lives of the people; and also, creating "State boards of health," before whom parties de-, siring to practice Medicine and Surgery should appear for examination, and obtain a certificate of qualification, and thus, by a higher standard of professional attainments enforced by legal enactments, have forced irresponsible ignorance of all pretended theories, to migrate to those states having no protective legislation.

It is a fact not to be denied, that there are Medical Schools in the United States whose faculties issue "diplomas" to irresponsible persons for a nominal sum, not requiring a prescribed period of study, or a certain qula-ification; or, who issue "bogus" diplomas of medicine, or law, purporting to have been issued by faculties of legally chartered "schools" of medicine, or law. And it is also a fact, (beyond contradiction), that there are agen-, encies in different parts of the west, known as "diploma brokers," who ad-vertise to furnish "diplomas" to persons in need of them, by means of which, they may evade the laws in force in those states prohibiting irres-ponsible persons from practicing Medicine and Surgery, which practice if permitted to continue, will be as destructive to the health and lives of the people as to place whisky, improved fire-arms, and amunition in the hands of an Indian.

All members of the profession (of every theory of practice,) who, if hon-est in their calling, are toiling more for the advancement of their science; the amelioration of suffering; the prevention of disease and the prolonga-, tion of life, than for hire; while the contrary will be the object and effect of the ignorant pretender.

Since there are a number of "medical schools, or universities," differing in theories, but in other essentials agreeing, and are unanimous in express-, ing their convictions, that the poorest "theory," if an educated one, is far better than the best, ignorantly applied in practice. The legitimate mem-bers of the profession, embracing every "theory of practice," are in favor of such legislation as will not discriminate against theory, but which will place each in the same balance, and suject all to the same tests; and there-, by raise the standard of the Medical Profession of this state, which will necessarily preserve and prolong the lives of the people.

PROCEEDINGS.

Society of Physicians and Surgeons of South-Western Iowa.

MURRAY, MARCH 5th, 1878.

Meeting called to order; Dr. Grigg presiding, with Dr. Nance, Secretary. Minutes of last meeting read and approved. Dr. Mauran, was admitted to membership. Dr. Torrey read an able paper on *Surgery.*

Dr. Mauran called attention to the frequent inequality of normal limbs.

Dr. Wilson referred to a report from the "American Medical Society," declaring that shortening in fractures of the long bones was the rule. Drs. Christie, Grigg, Nance, and Givin, coinciding.

Dr. Christie offered the following for discussion: "Is Pneumonia an essential fever? or is it a local inflammation."

Dr. Wilson stated that he considered it a local inflammation, and that the fever was symptomatic; often of malarial origin. For treatment, he gave cathartics, then relied entirely upon "Opium and Quinine." As a rule Pneumonia patients required but little treatment.

Dr. Christie understood the disease to be an essential fever; often assuming the epidemic form. He considered large doses of "Quinine," and moderate doses of "Opium," reliable treatment.

Dr. Lawrence was not prepared to say whether the disease was an essential fever, or symptomatic of the local inflammation; but that able clinical teachers classed the disease among the infectious. He thought the grave form, "Crupous Pneumonia" required other treatment than "Opium and Quinine." That where the bronchial secretion was of plastic, or rather a fibrinous exudation thrown out by the blood, as is the case with the disease occurring in Southern Ills. Mo. Ky. and Tenn., of which disease, most of the patients die. Such cases would be made worse in the first stage, by giving full doses of "Opium," in consequence of its paralyzing effect upon the epithelial structure of the capillary bronchial tubes, producing a dry condition of the mucous surface, with accumulations of inspissated secretion. He had noticed in the cases coming under his observation, that whenever he had controlled the circulation, and could get up profuse diaphoresis, a like moist condition of the mucous surfaces would follow, with lowering temperature, and certain relief to grave symptoms. A plethoric subject with "Crupous Pneumonia" in the first stage, he would rely upon "Venesection," Tart: Emetic, and Verat: Viride. As for Catarrhal Pneumonia, the form prevailing in Iowa, he con- sidered it simply a slight indisposition, depending upon exposure, and requiring but little treatment.

Dr. Mauran stated that his first experience was behind the lancet. He had seen it go down and rise again, only to disappear in the "dim distance." He thought the less treatment in pneumonia, the better for the patient.

Dr. Grigg thought that "Veratrum Viride," had justly taken the place of the lancet in the treatment of "Pneumonia."

Dr. Wilson said that the "blood and thunder" treatment originated years ago, because the pathology of the disease was not then understood, and had long since for good cause been abandoned.

In discussing Dr. Grigg's paper on "Materia Medica," Dr. Wilson said he considesed 15 to 40 gr. doses of "Hydrat Chloral" risky practice; and re- ferred to a Typhoid Fever patient having taken 80 grs. with impunity, but after some improvement in the patient, a 20 gr. dose produced alarming symptoms. He argued that where the powers of life are about exhausted, the drug would not enter the circulation, but would lay in the stomach as an inert substance. After improvement, smaller doses than had been giv- en, would be rapidly taken into the circulation, attended with alarming symptoms which might prove fatal.

Dr. Christie agreed with Dr. Wilson in giving small doses of the drug. He favored combining with Potassii Bromid., or with Morphia Sulph. In "Delirium Tremens" he thought large doses of the drug would be tolerated.

Dr. Mauran thought large doses of fresh "Chloral" was safe in compari- son to an old deliquesced article. He inquired whether the action of "Sal- icylic Acid" was not similar to that of "Quinine."

Dr. Christie referred to a case of "Rheumatism" which he had treated with "Colchicum, Iodid Pot. and Quinine," without benefit, but which was at once relieved by the "Salicylic Acid" treatment.

Dr. Roberts instanced a case of "Rheumatism" of malarial origin, treated with 40 grs. of "Quinine," without benefit, but which was relieved by the gradual introduction of 60 grs. of the "Acid."

Dr. Christie in discussing the subject of Dr. Roberts' paper, said that he believed "Diphtheria" to be first local, afterwards constitutional. The treatment should be "Antiseptic," first and last, with sustaining the patient.

Dr. Nance thought the disease constitutional, with local manifestations in the throat.

Dr. Wilson thought the disease at first local, afterwards constitutional, and that first local applications should be caustic.

Dr. Nance opposed caustic applications in any stage of the disease as producing shock to the patient. He would recommend ice locally, and also demulcent iced gargles.

Dr. Lawrence was opposed to the use of caustics, or any harsh procedure in any stage of the disease. That the strugglings of the patient interfered with a successful application of caustics, and that wounding, or abrasion of the healthy mucous membrane would be a sure consequence, upon which the exudation would attach, with increased facility for empoisonment by absorption of "Diphtheritic Virus." That grave cases could only be benefitted by treatment within the first 48 hours. That remedies should be used in the form of gargles or spray, which are sure destroyers of paracitic vegetations, and which will coagulate the exudation, thereby preventing organization of the false membrane; after which, garglings should be such as would disinfect and hasten the sloughing off of the false membrane, by encouraging the suppurative process. He opposed the use of ice, applications as retarding the (suppurative) process by which the false membrane is detached; as the longer the organized membrane adheres to the surface, the greater danger of empoisonment of the system. Since the disease terminates by "Asthenia." sustaining the powers of life should be a main feature of treatment. He was opposed to the use of Calomel, Mustard Plasters, and Blisters; or any application to the fauces that could not be tolerated in an inflamed eye; and especially condemning Tannic Acid, characterising it as the poorest application that had ever been tried, alleging that it simply produced a "Tannate" of the exudation, (or false membrane,) retarding the sloughing process, and thereby endangering the life of the patient.

The President revised the "Board of Censors," by appointing to fill vacancies, Drs. Lawrence, Howe, and Torrey.

The Society adjourned to meet at Creston, June 5th, 1878.

The foregoing report was written from hastily prepared notes by myself. It will be found in many respects to be inaccurate as to language used; the object being to state the position taken by those engaging in the discussion. If the position taken by any one has been incorrectly stated, it will be a pleasure for me to make the necessary corrections.—ED.

BOOKS AND PAMPHLETS RECEIVED.

The Cincinnati Lancet and Observer, for January 1878, J. C. CULBERT-
SON, M. D., Editor. T. M. STEVENS, M. D., of Indianapolis, Assistant Editor,
Published monthly by J. C. Culbertson, M. D., Cincinnati Ohio.

The American Medical Bi-Weekly for February 1878, E. S. GAILLARD,
M. D., Editor, Published Bi-Weekly by E. S. Gaillard, M. D., Louisville Kentucky.

The Pacific Medical and Surgical Journal, for February, and March,
1878, HENRY GIBBSONS, M. D. AND HENRY GIBBSONS, JR., M. D. Editors,
Published Monthly by Henry Gibbsons, M. D. and Henry Gibbsons, Jr.
M. D., San Francisco Cal.

*The American Journal of Obstetrics and Diseases of Women and Chil-
dren,* for January 1878. PAUL F. MUNDE, M. D., Editor, Published Quarterly by WM. Wood & Co., New York City.

The Medical Brief, for January, February, and March 1878, J. J. LAW-
RENCE, M. D., Editor, Published Monthly by Chas. E. Ware & Co., St.
Louis Mo.

ANNOUNCEMENT:—Spring Session 1878, of *The St. Louis Medical
College,* J. T. HODGEN, M. D., Dean of the Faculty of St. Louis Medical
College.

ANNUAL ANNOUNCEMENT:—Of *The Medical College of the Pacific,*
(Late Medical Department of the University of the Pacific,) Being the
"*Medical Department of University (City) College,*" San Francisco, Cal.
The Twentieth Regular Course Beginning June 3rd 1878, and ending in
October, HENRY GIBBSONS, JR M. D., Dean.

BOOK NOTICE.

Ziemssen's 'Cyclopedia of the Practice of Medicine, DR. H. VON ZIEMSSEN,
Editor; WM. WOOD & co., New York City, Publishers of the American
Edition. E. G. Taber, Oskaloosa Iowa, Agent for Iowa, and Nebraska.

We have seen several volumes of this excellent work, which contain
the Medical Literature of the world on each subject treated. If the remaining numbers compare with those issued, no Physician, or Medical
Student should be without this "complete work."

CⱯTHEⱭⱭ

IOWA CATLIN.

Vol. I.—MAY, 1878.—No. II.

Original Communication.

Ethics, Professional Ethics.

Extract from an Essay, By W. H. Christie, M, D., Read Before
the Society of Physician's and Surgeons of South-Western
Iowa, at Murrray, March 5th 1878,

Mr. Chairman, and Gentleman:—Will you doubt my pro-
bity, or my correctness when I say that the conduct of the majority of medical men outside of the beneficial influence of
Medical Societies to one another, is absolutely piratical and
damnable, and as destitute of morality as the Chinese are of
virtue; and who practice the precepts of the Golden rule,
"Do unto others as you would have them do unto you," about
as frequently as Bob. Ingersoll asks a blessing.   How different then the hopes we have as young men leaving Medical

College, instilled with pure and noble motives from the instruction of a "Proud Alma Mater," and swinging our shingle to the breeze, we anxiously sit and wait to be called to a case. Finally we are summoned to see "some old Granny," who, perhaps has survived her usefulness, and has taken medicine—Single—Double—Combined, and probably every heterogeneous combination of infernal mixture.

Now the Young Doctor, the latest addition to the faculty, is called to give his wisdom a chance. With fear and trembling he approaches the shrunken form of withered humanity. No hope to give, but a speedy removal from this vale of tears.

However, he must do something. He gives his opinion that ere long, she will depart unto her fathers, and that he can do nothing more than soothe the way that leads hence.

The old Doctor is informed of what the young Doctor said; he has his friends—Satellites; why should he not have them! See the curl on his lip as he sneeringly says, "what does he know about the matter?" "He has never practiced medicine!" And he will further say, "that if she takes his medicine she will die."

The Young Doctor learns of his senior's remarks through a reliable source. Of course he feels happy. He solemnly swears that he will fight it out on that line, if it takes a decade. With zealous indiscretion he permits his feelings gradually to become embittered toward the senior practitioner, who conducts himself in such a manner as to give the junior reason to think, and understand, that (he) the senior, has a "cutthroat" mortgage upon the business of that town, and that (he) the junior is trespassing upon "encumbered" territory.

Junior considers this to be a free country; "grab to be the game," and he solemnly swears, that the first opportunity offered he will make senior think that an "attachment" is about to issue.

The time has arrived. The old Doctor has a rush of business. There is an "hysterical" female, who, during an indisposition has been left alone for a few hours, when a thunder storm breaks forth, with its first angry explosion, disturbing peace which reigned within, by raising the hair on the sick ladys head, as well as raising "satanas." The nurse returning after her usual gossip, and finds the lady in terrible convulsions.

Being the only one to be found, the Young Doctor is called; he rushes into the room and seating himself near the patient, commences an examination with more airs than "Æsculapius," wisely remarking—terrible convulsion—irritation at the base of the brain. Relapsing into deep meditation, he no doubt determines to use a vigorous effort to supplant "satanas" this hitch.

Soon the patient revives, exclaiming, Oh! How much better I feel—Doctor do give to me another dose of that medicine! It seems to be just what I need. Oh Dear! My heart flutters so!

The Doctor assures her that she has been very ill, and he proceeds to make a thorough examination of the case. He listens to that heart, without a Stethoscope, (but it is not always necessary to have one; to create a favorable impression.) Placing his left hand gently upon her side, percusses the chest. In response to questions asked, she says she has pain in the top of her head, of a burning character. The whole chain of uterine symptoms are recited, and after a careful review of them, the Doctor inquires of the patient whether she had been treated locally, for uterine disease, to which she answered "No." Well Madam, that is the trouble with you; uterine disease, and it has been made worse by improper treatment. You need not expect to get relief, without receiving correct treatment. There has been wonderful improvement in the Gynæcological department of medical science within the last few years. The older physicians follow too much a routine of practice, and handle these cases much as they did 20 years ago.

All present are amazed at the fluency with which he converses. So young in years, yet so ripe in knowledge. His professional stock on the market is "bulled," while the old doctor's is "beared," correspondingly.

The young doctor is even. The old doctor trys to get "evener," and henceforth, they keep up a perpetual fight, until we find that they have about a mutual respect and hatred for one another.

Now this is about the conduct of physicians competing for practice, who acknowledge no restraint, by reason of ethics.

Having organized a medical society for the purpose of correcting irregularities, ungentlemanly asperities, barbarism, and piracy, do we propose to do it, or do we intend to be a body of mere pretenders, and thus imitate a quack, the lowest and meanest order of created intelligence?

How much have we advanced in professional honor, as members of the Society of Physicians and Surgeons of South-Western Iowa, than we should have, had we not organized as such. In order to determine, let us consider its object. 1. To promote advancement in Medical Science, by united co-operation, in which the truly meritorious can descern a reward for his efforts. 2. United we are better enabled to protect legitimate Medicine, and to more strongly define it, not only to ourselves, but exhibit it to the public in contrast with "Quackery." 3. The spirit of the American Code of Medical Ethics is such, that all true Physicians are required to stand upon their own merits.

"It is derogatory to the dignity of the profession, to resort to public advertisements, or private cards or hand-hills inviting the attention of individuals affected with particulr diseases. To publicly offer advice and medicine to the poor, gratis. To promise radical cures. To publish cases and operations in the public prints, or suffer such publication to be made. To invite laymen to be present to witness operations. To boast of cures, and remedies. To adduce certificates of skill and success, or to perform any other similar acts: These being the ordinary practices of empirics, are highly reprehensible in a regular physician.

General rules should be adopted by the faculty in every town, or district, relative to pecuniary acknowledgements from their patients, and it should be deemed a point of honor, to adhere to them with as much uniformity as varying circumstances will admit."

How much better, or more dignified, is the medical profession (in these parts) than the 'vociferating clam-boy,' or the cheap boot-black? It is true our abdomen may be more rotund from better living, our clothes may fit more neatly, and that we may assume to be gentlemen of professional standing because of these characters, which however are but thin shells covering up a dangerous fraud.

That we may advance in Science, we should deal with our brother as such, avoiding discourtesies. To be guarded in casting reflections upon his character. This may be hard to avoid, but here is our tribunal, and here we plead our cause, honestly, fearlessly; and let this be the end, so long as parties comply with the code of ethics,; but deal strenuously regardless of whom, whenever found deviating from a course of professional rectitude. Only in the discharge of this duty, can peace and harmony exist in our midst. We will then be respected by the public, and we will have respect for our professional brother. Until such relation be established and maintained, can we hope for advancement in medical science? Or for Professional Honor?

[We regret very much our inability to publish this article in full as read before the Society, owing to its extreme length. Having made as correct an extract, as its length and and attendant circumstances would permit, we trust the author will be correctly represented by it.—Ed.]

True Animal Vaccination.

By Henry A. Martin, M. D,, of Boston, Mass.

My attention has been called to the article on vaccination by Dr. Agard, and your editorial remarks thereon, in your issue for October, 1877. Although your opinions are entirely in accordance with the spirit of Dr. Agard's paper and opposed to animal vaccination, I cannot doubt that both your wishes and his is to arrive at truth; nor do I believe that having opened your columns to an opponent of animal vaccination you will close them to a very ardent and decided advocate of that innovation. Pregnant, as it must be, for good or evil, I therefore offer for publication an answer to Dr. Agard, as brief as is consistent with anything like a fair presentation of my case.

Before proceeding to answer Dr. Agard, it may be proper for me to inform your readers who I am and what claim I may be supposed to have to being considered an authority on vaccination, and, above all, on animal vaccination. This is peculiarly necessary in a discussion with an adversary who, while professing no special knowledge of his topic, brings forward such a formidable and imposing display of world-renowned "authorities."

"Truth is mighty and will prevail." If I did not fully believe this I should hardly venture, armed with nothing but a few positive and absolutely ascertained facts, to go forth against the serried ranks of Von Hebra, Seaton, Simon, and others, skillfully led by Dr. Agard. The personal introduction and narrative I offer is, in every way, the fittest preface and corrollary to what I have to say, and, indeed, is absolutely necessary to a clear comprehension of the force of my argument. Therefore, without further apology, I must state that I am a pretty old practitioner, having taken a diploma as M. D. at Harvard in 1845. From the commencement of my student life I took a very peculiar interest in the subject of vaccination, and when I entered on practice, gave a very unusual amount of attention to its practice, for which there was an ample field in the prodigious number of unvaccinated children at that time. Very soon after I commenced practice I became aware of the extremely precarious and unreliable supply of vaccine virus, and that there was no State provision, as in other countries, for such supply; that the only sources from which the profession derived virus were the dispensaries of New York and the office of the city physician in Boston, and, perhaps, in other large cities. The virus procured from these sources was from the very poorest and most squalid classes, in which would be the greatest likelihood, if anywhere, of the existence of the unfortunate inheritors of ancestral vice and disease. This virus was, for the most part, collected by medical students and young physicians who had no special knowledge of vaccination nor any interest in it save for the trifling pecuniary return from the sale of the virus. In the whole length and breadth of the United States there did not exist any State provision for the supply of vaccine virus, nor any private source worthy of any reliance whatever. I am sure your older readers will corroborate this assertion.

About the year 1850 some cases of small-pox occurred in a crowded perlieu of the suburb of Boston. It was necessary that I should vaccinate some twenty or more quite unprotected children in the neighborhood. I had no virus. I went to the city physician of Boston and purchased, for two dollars, twenty quill points. With these I "vaccinated," very carefully, twenty children without result. This process was repeated five times, without success in any single instance. Each new lot of twenty points had to be paid for, for at that time the doctrine held by the dignitaries who condescended to sell so-called "vaccine virus," was that it was so perishable an article that warranting its efficacy was a thing out of the question. I then wrote to New York, and from the complement of three lots of ten points each, had one successful result, that is one case in which two vesicles appeared, went through a course very familiar to the admirers of long-humanized virus, but very different, indeed, from that described and returned by Jenner, Willan, Nyce, Coxe and the other numerous early and only true authorities on what vaccination should be and was before it reached the lowest degree of deterioration. Poor as was the development of "vaccinia" from this New York virus, I hailed it joyfully and hoped, by careful "culture," to bring it up in quality.

I made several inoculations with virus from the most perfect, or rather the least imperfect of the two vesicles; every one of them failed. There was at that time a firm of French druggists in New York, C. A. Patusel & Co., who advertised "cow-pox virus from the French Academy of Medicine" in capillary tubes. In my distress I sent for some of these, and having perfectly ascertained that they were from the vaccine department of the Academy, I made several vaccinations with their contents. The result was admirable, the most vigorous, typically perfect development of "vaccinia" I had ever seen, the finest I have ever yet seen, excepting only from vaccination from the animal. Nothing could be better in the way of humanized virus, and, long after, I ascertained that this French lymph was of a very early human remove from original cow-pox. The progress of the vaccinations made with this virus corresponded very exactly with that described and figured by the earliest writers on vaccination. The "vesicle" was so full and perfect in form, and the "areola" so intense and wide, that I never attempted to produce more than two, and, in infants, often not more than one vesicle. The phenomena accompanying the development of even a single vesicle, the engorgement of the axillary glands, the feeble reaction on the ninth, tenth and eleventh days, all described by the earlier vaccinators and all insisted upon by them as absolutely necessary to a protective vaccination, were so different from what people were accustomed to as sometimes to excite alarm.

Nothing, however, could be less called for. All the vaccinations made with this virus were, in every way, in every part of the process, to the invariable formation of a crust of typical form, consistence and color, all that could be desired.

I was delighted with my success, and for four years, during which I vaccinated over 1500 patients, I used this and nothing else. At the end of that time I unfortunately lost it, sent again to New York, obtained several new lots of tubes, but was never able to recover the treasure I had lost. I then went into correspondence with the National Vaccine Institution of England, and various other institutions and individuals in Europe. After fully testing the supplies of lymph I obtained from these, I at last elected to propagate the "stock," of the first named only, as the very best virus of long-humanization of which I had then or have ever since had any conizance. A great many times I received from that noble Institution renewals of my stock, of this virus, perfect in its kind, and I shall never forget or fail to acknowledge the obligation. For a great many years, although I had and used, to a certain extent, many different "strains" of vaccine virus, I propagated and issued this almost exclusively.

I am, however, "getting before my story." In 1854 I delivered, before a local society, a paper "On Certain Points Connected with Vaccination and Revaccination." When I had read this paper I said that I knew the general difficulty which country physicians had to keep up a supply of vaccine virus; that I was continually vaccinating, and almost always had virus to spare, and would be happy to send a point or two to any gentleman who would send me his name and address, with a stamp to pay return postage. The result of this in three years, was that I often received from a dozen to twenty requests weekly to send virus to applicants, and more than half these applications were unaccompanied by a stamp. I had involved myself in a very responsible, troublesome, thankless, unprofitable, and indeed, expensive business. It occurred to me that if I put an advertisement into the *Medical Journal*, offering to do for remuneration what I had for three years been doing for nothing, I might be of service to the profession and the public; might possibly build up a business that would remunerate me for inevitably great labor and be of incalculable advantage in a country so wofully destitute of reliable means of vaccine supply. At any rate, if I should fail to accomplish all this, the plan opened a way for me to get rid of a great and unnecessary annoyance by referring applicants to my advertisement. I consulted a great many of the wisest and best men, the then leaders of the profession, and all, without exception, approved the plan and urged me to carry it out, saying that there was nothing unprofessional in it; that, on the contrary, if I succeeded. I should merit the very highest applause and gratitude of the profession and people of America. During that long period (since 1857) I have devoted an amount of labor to this specialty of vaccine supply and to the study of vaccination in all its possible relations, that given to any of the other and more brilliant and attractive fields of medical effort, could hardly have failed to bring me reward, in honor, distinction and fortune, which, as yet, I lack. If I never succeed in winning such reward, which many men gain for infinitely less effort, I have the very consolatory consciousness of having been the means, both before and since I introduced into America the method of true animal vaccination, of having done and been the means of there having been done an amount of good simply incalculable. I may never get the credit and applause for which I have so constantly labored, but I am, by no means, without hope of this, which is, after all, of very secondary importance.

During the years from 1857 to 1870, inclusive, I issued an annual average of 25,000 charged points, or their equivalent in other forms, of humanized virus. In 1864 a good deal of interest was felt in the introduction of the Italian method of animal vaccination into Paris, and, in this way, to the notice

of the general European profession. This introduction of a
method into general notice, which had been practiced in Naples and other Italian cities since 1810, was due to an address
on the subject made by Dr. Palasciano, of Naples, at the Medical Congress at Lyons in 1864. A young Dr. Lanoix was
present, heard the address, and as a result, went to Naples and
learned the Neapolitan method of vaccination from Dr. Negri,
a noted practitioner there, and the direct successor of its orig-
inator, Dr. Galbiati. With a heifer inoculated by Dr. Nigri,
Lanoix went to Paris and began his remarkable career as vaccinator. This Neapolitan method of vaccination, whatever
may have been *said* or written of it, was *not true* animal vaccination, but a very different thing, viz: Retro-vaccination, the
inoculation of a bovine animal with humanized virus, with a
view to restoring enfeebled virus to its prestine vigor, of purg-
ing contaminated virus from its impurity. It had been am-
ply and perfectly proved that it does neither, long, very long,
before 1864, by the famous Robert Ceely, and many other accurate and reliable observers, among the last and least of whom
was the Writer of this paper, nearly twenty-five years since.
D. Galbiati, in 1810, was lead to practice retro-vaccination
from having seen two undoubted cases of *vaccino-syphilis*,
and hit upon the idea of passing the Neapolitan vaccine virus
through the sytem of the cow and so purify it. This was precisely the same practice as that brought to the notice of the
Massachusetts Medical Society, some twenty or more years
ago by Dr. Cutter, of Woburn (near Boston); the same practiced by his son, Dr. Ephraim Cutter, to whom Dr. Agard al-
ludes in very complimentary terms, as a source of an enormous number of "scabs" supplied to the United States army and
to others for many years before 1870, and, to a limited extent,
after that year.

It is not necessary for me to say anything more about retro-
vaccination, except that Boisquet, Ceely, and a host of others
of the higher authorities, have decided that by retro-vaccina-

tion enfeebled human vaccinia cannot be restored, nor contaminated virus purified.   My own repeated experiments and observations confirm these prominent authorities; but if further evidence is wanting of the worthlessness of retro-vaccination and of the virus so obtained, it can be furnished in quite overwhelming amount by the experience in its use in our army in 1863–4, and of many hundreds of physicians who have employed it.   The obstacle to the reception and adoption of *true* animal vaccination, resulting from the worthlessness of the virus of retro-vaccination, was, beyond all others, the greatest. In April, 1866, the ever-famous cases of original cow-pox at Beaugency, (near Orleans, in France), was reported to the Vaccine Committee of the French Academy of Medicine, of which Professior Depaul was the head *Directeur de la Vaccine.*

The story of the visit of Prof. Depaul and others of the vaccine committee to Beaugency, the solemn *proces verbal*, to verify every step of the process, and the transportaion of the sacred heifer, inoculated with the precious treasure to Paris, and "a little building in the garden of the Academy," is an interesting one.   I have told it once in print, and it will soon appear at greater length again from my pen.   I will not attempt to relate it here, although many a ponderous volume has been devoted to events and transactions of infinitely less importance to mankind—present and future.

With Dr. Depaul, the heifer of Beaugency and an annual appropriation of 6,000 francs, began, in 1866, the practice of *true* animal vaccination, to-wit: The inoculation of a selected young animal of the bovine species, from this another, and so on, in endless series as a source, and the only source, of virus for human vaccination. This it is of which I am an humble but ardent advocate.   The introduction of that method into America, and far more than this, the constant labor to vindicate it through good and evil report, against the attacks of stupidity, ignorance, and more than either, of superficial students, not of vaccination, but of a vast literature, the good of which they have not recognised, nor rejected the worthless, is the one claim on which rests my humble but confident hope to some grateful remembrance among men when I shall have gone *ad majorum.* I was, of course, very much interested in all this matter of Lanoix and Depaul, and should have gone to Paris, personally, to investigate it all, but could not get away from pressing and multifarious engagements. From 1866 to 1870, I was constantly receiving letters of inquiry about animal vaccination. To these, and there were full two hundred of them, I invariably answered that I had no real and practical knowledge of the subject; that I had read all that was accessible, and that my opinion, based on this reading (chiefly English publications) and on my own experience in retro-vaccination, was decidedly that it would prove of no value or vitality, and that I had not the slightest idea of ever abandoning the admirable virus of the English Vaccine Institution for the result of the innovation. This was my very sincere opinion. I suppose Dr. Seaton was at the bottom of my prejudice against even true animal vaccination.

During 1869 and the early part of 1870, I had letters of introduction to our Minister at Paris, and to leaders of the profession there, and hoped from month to month to go there, but at last had to give up that project and send a most trustworthy agent, who was familiar with my views and wishes, to Paris to gather all possible literature and information in regard to animal vaccination, and to bring ample supplies of virus. This agent returned on September 23, 1870, and on that day I inoculated three heifers with virus from Professor Depaul's 258th, 259th and 260th animals, by the method recommended in autograph directions from that very noble and eminent, but most shamefully maligned and inadequately appreciated man. On following days I vaccinated others, and in every instance, with success. From that time till now I have been a constant observer of the effects of true animal vaccination, and through the correspondence of over 9,000 physicians, of all schools, who have been supplied with virus from my stables, the recipient of the results of the observation and experience of others. During more than seven years since the autumn of 1870, virus directly from the animal, to vaccinate over 1,000,000 of human beings, has been issued by my cow and myself. Scores, perhaps hundreds, of physicians have, to a greater or less extent, practiced the vaccination of animals with a view to supplying virus to the profession. Some of these have done this to a very large extent. Among these I may mention Dr. Foster, of New York, my first follower in this field; Dr. Griffin of Fon du Lac, Wisconsin, both of these with virus and instruction from myself, and Dr. Kuseny, of Chambersburg, Pennsylvania, who started with virus from Dr. Griffin. All of these gentlemen have distributed very large amounts of true animal virus of excellent quality.

The result of all this competition and labor of so many physicians has been the entire revolutionizing of vaccination in America. During the last seven years many millions have been vaccinated *directly* from the animal. An epidemic of quite unprecedented malignity in the memory of the living, has occurred during those years, and this has led to the general and public vaccination of cities and towns with a rapidity and effect impossible before the practice of animal vaccination, and quite unknown before in America or even Europe. Even the gentlemen like Dr. Davis, Dr. Agard and yourselves, who still oppose animal vaccination, are reaping its benefits in the use of virus of but a few human removes from the cow, which it is quite possible is, to all practical intents, as protective as that purely animal, and is, at any rate, a very different and other thing from the very long humanized virus which was in use in England before the Estlin cow-pox in 1832; in France before the Passy and Rambouillet cow-pox in 1836, and in San Francisco in 1868–9, before the introduction of true animal vaccination and the Beaugency virus in

September, 1870. A great many of the most voluble opponents of true vaccination have never used anything else than early removes from it, and know nothing really of the peculiarities of long-humanized virus, for it is not probable that a particle of vaccine virus exists in the United States but that from the animal or of early human removes therefrom.

Dr. Agard makes some mistakes, as, for instance, in stating that Dr. Depaul went to Italy in 1864 and introduced animal vaccination into Paris. It was Dr. Lanoix, and he introduced the Neapolitan method of retro-vaccination. Professor Depaul introduced *true* animal vaccination in 1866, and did not go to Italy at all. He also states that his friend Dr. Cutter has had by far the largest experience of any man in America in cow-pox vaccination, when the vast mass, if not all that gentleman's experience, is of retro-vaccination, and of the effect of its resulting virus, must be very limited; at all events there are certainly many men in America, beside myself, who have had infinitely larger experience in cow-pox vaccination. Dr. Agard seems also to entirely confound true animal vaccination with retro-vaccination, a most common mistake, and which has given a very unfortunate impression in regard to the former. I will not, however, dilate on these errors of doctor Agard, natural and excusable in a writer who does not relate his personal observation and experience, but writes from a laborious and studious compilation of "Authorities." Of these he has brought forward a formidable array, so formidable that nothing but the perfect annihilation of animal vaccination and of the few humble American partisans thereof who care to write with anything but the vaccine point in the, arms of their patients, was to be looked for.

Dr. Agard may, however, rest assured that animal vaccination will survive and prosper, notwithstanding the tremendous artillery of big names which Prof. *N. S. Davis*, of Cincinnati, has so industriously loaded to the muzzle, and doctor Agard, of California, fired off at second-hand with a great display of scientific erudition.

It is asserted by the advocates of *true* animal vaccination that: 1. It is *proved* that the casual inoculation of *adults* (the dairy people of Gloucestershire and elsewhere, before 1798), with the virus of original cow-pox, is absolutely and perfectly protective from small-pox, for the rest of life, in precisely the same way and degree that a first attack of small-pox, *in adult life*, is absolutely and perfectly protective from a second attack.

2. It is *not proved* that the intentional inoculation of even an adult, with the virus of original and spontaneously occurring cow-pox is absolutely and perfectly protective, in like manner; for there have been few such inoculations, and no record of them exist. But it is *assumed* that perfect protection would be afforded by the inoculation of an adult with such virus.

3. It is *proved* that even primary adult vaccination with humanized lymph is not absolutely and perfectly protective from small-pox for the rest of life, while primary vaccination of infants with lymph of *long* humanization can hardly be said to be any protection of the individual, after adult age, from the *occurrence* of small-pox, though it certianly does, in a great proportion of cases, exercise a decided modifying power on the gravity and fatality of such post-vaccinal attacks of *variola.*

4. Although cases of small-pox, after adult primary vaccination with humanized virus were noticed and recorded very soon after the introduction of vaccination, they were so rare as to be easily accounted for by the imperfection and spuriousness of the vaccination.

5. These cases prior to 1823 (the year of Jenner's death), although numerous in the aggregate, still bore so small a proportion to the sum of all those who had been vaccinated as not seriously to shake the popular and professional confidence in vaccination. The confidence of the people and of the profession in Jenner was so great that during his life his confi-

dent assurances, and more or less ingenious and plausible explanations were accepted. After his death, however, the occurrence of post vaccinal variola became so frequent as to make new theories absolutely necessary, to explain their occurrence. It was at this time that Dr. Gregory began (in the London *Medical Gazette*), the annual publication of statistics of the great Small-pox Hospital in his charge. The statement that over twenty per cent, of his patients bore on their persons the distinct marks or cicatrices of a single vaccination, created something like a panic. These returns, made each year since Gregory began them, now show a percentage of over ninety (90) such cases. At this time began the practice of re-vaccinations, admitted at first by the most faithful Jennerites as a test to ascertain whether the subject had been really vaccinated properly, or a means of replacing or restoring the protection lost or impaired by the lapse of time and mysterious changes in the system, by those less sure of the unchangeable permanence of protection afforded by the most primary vaccination.

6. It is absolutely proved that certain changes are observed in the phenomena of vaccinia as it is more and more removed from its original source by successive and numerous human transmissions. These changes are seen in a very slow and gradual, but constant diminution of the length of the period from the insertion of virus to appearance and development of areola, and from that till fall of crust; a great diminution in the vividness and extent of the areola, a diminution and, at last, entire absence of the enlargement of the glands in the axilla, and of that reactive fever invariably noticed and insisted upon by Jenner as a proof of constitutional effect, and a *sine qua non* of protective vaccination.

7. These very great changes are not the result of passing through a single human system; but the very gradual result of the transmission of a disease purely animal in its origin through a long series of exotic (human) systems.

8. It is assumed that the diminution of protection afforded by an adult vaccination, or even an adult re-vaccination, from what was noticed during the first twenty years of vaccination, must be due to a diminution of the protective efficacy of the vaccinia induced by virus weakened by very long and frequently repeated humanization; at any rate, it is claimed that it is sufficiently probable that the diminution of the intensity of the vaccinia, induced by long humanized virus, is associated with a great diminution in its protective value and efficacy, for us to endeavor, if possible, to obtain vaccine virus which shall be as intense and may be as prophylactic in its effects as that casually received on the hands of the milkers of Gloucestershire, whose perfect and permanent protection thereby is the one solid rock and basis of the doctrine of vaccination.

9. The virus we want, to fully and locally meet the requirements of the need in which we are placed by the change in the vaccine disease by long humanization, is, of course, the virus of original, spontaneously occurring cow-pox. This not being a thing that can be obtained except at long and quite uncertain intervals, we are led to an experiment so natural and scientific that nothing but a familiarity with the history of vaccination, its early hopes, enthusiasms and confidence, can explain to us why there ever was any other mode practiced of perpetuating original cow-pox—the experiment of inoculating with the virus of original spontaneously occurring cow-pox in the cow, a selected young animal of the same species. If we find that virus obtained from one such artificial bovine transmission induces precisely the same symptoms in the human subject as the use of the original virus, we shall have gained some ground for confidence in true animal vaccination.

If, after there have been at least five hundred *successive* bovine transmissions of original disease, we find that virus from the five hundredth heifer, after nearly twelve years' separation from the original case, induces on the human arm an eruption exactly in the two infinitely important points of duration and reactive fever, identical with that from the first, we may have great confidence that *true* animal vaccination is a great, infinitely important and beneficial innovation in practice. Such is my firm opinion, and that the universal adoption of the virus obtained by the exclusively bovine transmission of original cow-pox is only a question of time.

The success of the innovation has been wonderful in America, when we reflect that it is due to nothing but a deep-seated and well founded belief that, in a return to its animal source was to be found the only remedy for the defects in the prophylaxy of vaccination, the only escape from the possible horror which some medical philosophers and statisticians think so slight a matter, of syphilitic contamination. If one man in a million gets syphilized, or has his baby syphilized by vaccination, it is a very small item for the medical or statistical quidnunc, but a very large one for the man or his baby.

In your brief editorial note you intimate a belief that the profession is inclined to abandon the use of animal virus. I am utterly at a loss to understand upon what data this intimation may be based. If you live ten years (as I hope you may a thousand) and exercise your usual acuteness of observation, you will be aware of the fact that the career of true animal vaccination is barely commencing, not ended or nearly so. That it should have accomplished what it has, in spite of all able opposition of men officially bound and pledged to oppose it *"talibus et unguis"* is a perfect proof of its vitality and value. *Magna est veritas et prevalebit.* If true animal vaccination is founded on truth, it will prevail, despite the laborious compilations of Davis and his disciples. If false, it will fall, even without such opposition, and I will be the first to say Amen.

I have alluded to only one and the most important argument, in my mind, in favor of true animal vaccination, viz., the superiority of the prophylaxy it affords. There are others to four of which I will briefly allude:

  1. The entire immunity of true animal vaccine virus from all possibility of being the vehicle of syphilis or other *human* disease. The reports of transmission of *animal* disease, except cow-pox, are simply, and *without exception*, false, and can only be credited by those who are utterly ignorant of the phenomena of vaccination in the heifer. The "two cases of Charbon, following animal vaccination, in *England*," never had any existence, save in the fertile and mendacious mind of M. Jules Guerin. It would take too long to relate how M. Guerin originally reported those cases *himself* to *l'Union Medicale*, for April, 1873, as of Charbon, following animal vaccination in *New* England; and how, when he found that Charbon is a disease unknown in (North), America he shifted the scene to England. The foundation for any report of such cases was the death of two old adults, at Falmouth, Massachusetts, who were vaccinated, each from a different crust of *humanized* virus, and afterwards exposed to severe and protracted cold, and, as a consequence of that exposure, died, from seven to ten days after vaccination. The virus was used in a very large number of other cases, with nothing but regular and beneficial results. The cases were reported as following true animal vaccination, and are the only cases so reported except one, very recently, in the *New York Medical Record*, Dec. 22d, in regard to which an article from my pen will probably appear in that journal. After infinite labor I obtained evidence, which I have in letters from, 1 the reporter; 2, the vaccinator; and 3, the person who supplied the virus, that the virus employed in these cases of "Charbon" was, in both instances, humanized. I have never yet refuted in the *Boston Medical and Surgical Journal*, Jan. 23d, 1873, because I did not procure all the evidence till very lately, neither did I think it worth while to do so till lately I discovered that the two Falmouth cases were M. Guerin's two cases of Charbon in *England*. Soon I shall tell the whole

story, is for no other reason, to show how such controversalists as **M**. Guerin manufacture and "cook their facts."

2. The advantages of unlimited supply of virus, afforded by proper performance of animal vaccination, in times of epidemic and panic, and the avoidance thereby of "vaccine famines," such as that which has recently been experienced in England, and loudly and bitterly complained of in almost every medical journal, through the whole of the epidemic, despite the enormously expensive governmental arrangement for vaccine supply.

3. The security, from the production of true animal virus by men of a certain amount of special knowledge, and the escape thereby from the infinite and miserable malpractice resulting from the collection of virus from imperfect and spurious vesicles, and at improper periods of the disease, and the consequent production of an entirely unprotective disease, by the ignorant and unprincipled men who are occasionally found with a post normal **M. D.**

4. The perfect immunity of true animal vaccination from erysipelas, that "pest of the vaccinator"—for not one case of erysipelas has been hitherto reported—partly to be ascribed to vaccination with true animal virus; and only two cases in which there could possibly have been even a suspicion of such complication; a suspicion which the slighest investigation dissipated at once.

These advantages, and others, are so clear and indubitable, that argument on them would be idle.

In case any of my readers feel disposed to further investigate the subject of animal vaccination, I may refer them to a long report, by myself, on animal vaccination, which will appear, very soon, in the forthcoming volume of the *Transactions of the American Medical Association.*

In throwing together these remarks on true animal vaccination, I have made no display of "authorities;" but if **Dr.** Agard, or anybody else, is disposed to dispute the accuracy of

any assertion I have made, he may be assured that ample
and perfect authority can and will be cited for every assertion. The really valuable authorities on animal vaccination
are not the very eminent men whom Dr. Davis and Dr.
Agard have quoted so liberally; men who have literally no
experience in true animal vaccination—but those who are not
only thoroughly familiar with the phenomena from vaccination with virus of long humanization, but with that from the
vaccination of animals and of the human subject with true
bovine lymph; and who are at the same time perfectly familiar with the history, literature and statistics of vaccination
since 1798. There are not many such authorities, and what
few there are, who might have a claim to be so considered,
have been very busy for the greater part of the past seven
years, in a much more important work than that of writing
laborious essays in defense of a method, the all-sufficient defense of which will surely be found in the result of the millions of vaccinations they have made in America with true animal virus. In my opinion, as true as one day follows another,
it will be found that the vaccination and re-vaccination, made
by this method during the past seven years in America, will
prove to be prophylactic from variolous disease, to a degree
never before known in the history of vaccination. To this
hoped-for result the believers in true animal vaccination look
forward with confidence; and with ample experience of the
infinitely slight effect of the most elaborate and learned arguments to convince any one "against his will," are willing
to waive an addition to their already onerous labors.—*Pacific Medical and Surgical Journal.*

[Having had no practical experience with *true animal*
vaccination, but have witnessed many failures and bad results
with the use of humanized virus, both in civil and military
practice. Because of positive and safe results, the *animal*
virus, or an early remove is to be preferred to that of long
humanized.—Ed.]

Sterility and its Treatment.

BY WILLIAM H. WATHEN, M. D., Clinical Lecturer on Diseases of
Women and Children, Louisville Medical College, Surgeon to the
Female Department, Louisville City Hospital.

As there are several interesting papers to be presented at
this meeting of our Association, I shall detain you but a few
minutes, and respectfully ask your attention to some remarks
on those forms of sterility that require surgical treatment.
To those who have neglected the study of this subject it
might not appear very practical; but when we reflect that
about every eighth marriage is barren, we see the necessity
of investigating every thing that can elucidate this important matter, especially since it is a fact that, clinically speaking, sterility does not, except in rare cases, denote the absolute impossibility of conception, but only the presence of a
greater or less obstacle.

Let us pass by the theories explaining the physiology of
conception, and assume that impregnation can only occur
when the living spermatozoa of the male come in contact with
the healthy ovule of the female, and that this must take place
within the uterus or fallopian tubes or on the ovaries, and
that where there is any thing to prevent this contact we invariably have sterility.

The causes that oppose the union of these two elements
are generally some congenital or acquired abnormal condition
of the female generative organs, and are seldom removed except by surgical interference. We shall confine our remarks
to this part of the subject, as it is imperfectly understood by
the general practitioner, who can devote but little time to
its study.

Most physicians are so accustomed to treat sterility consti-
tutionally that they are supposed to be quite familiar with
what we would term the constitutional and general causes,
such as sexual frigidity, syphilis, general debility, and ana-

mia, or the condition the opposite to that present in anæmia; that, namely, of over-feeding and luxurious habits, corpulency; and are fully capable of managing such cases intelligently and scientifically.

The abnormal conditions of the female organs referred to consist of mechanical obstructions in any part of the passages from the vulva to the fimbriated extremeties of the fallopian tubes, such as to interfere with the proper transit of the spermatic fluid or of the ovules. These obstructions may be considered in the following order:

(1) *Obstructions at the vulva or ostium vaginæ;*

(2) *Obstructions within the vagina;*

(3) *Obstructions at the os externum or within the cervical canal;*

(4) *Obstructions from malformation or displacement of the cervix;*

(5) *Obstructions from displacement of the uterus.*

It will be necessary to include under these headings those cases in which the vagina is incapable of retaining the semen, though, logically speaking, such a condition does not constitute an obstruction.

(1) *Obstructions of the Vulva or Ostium Vaginæ.*—When excessive development of the labia vulvæ, or hypertrophic or cancerous enlargement of clitoris, is an obstacle to intercourse and a cause of sterility, excision is indicated and may be safely performed. The hymen sometimes deviates from its normal crescent-shape, and partially or completely closes the entrance into the vagina, and prevents the introduction of the male organ. We usually have infertility with this deformity; but cases of impregnation are recorded where the semen was deposited only on the external parts of the female. By a physical examination we can readily detect the obstruction, and by crucial incisions can quickly and safely remove it.

Vaginismus always produces dyspareunia, and in most in-

stances an inability for sexual intercourse, and thereby frequently entails sterility. When it is the result of disease of
the uterus or its appendages, the treatment should be directed to the cause; but if simply a hyperæsthesia of the hymen
or vulvar outlet, we shall have to resort to other means. Until recently such cases baffled the skill of our profession, but
thanks to the genius of Sims, we can now insure these patients a perfect cure, and not only save them the mortifica-
tion of living without issue, but enable them to perform the
obligations of the marriage state. Having your patient ether-
ized and on her back or left side, seize the hymenial membrane (or its remains) with the tenaculum forceps at its
junction with the urethra, and with a pair of curved scissors
cut it all away in one continuous piece. In a few days the
cut surface is entirely healed and the operation for a radical
cure may be performed. This consists in making a deep incision through the vaginal tissue on each side of the mesial
line, beginning half an inch above the sphincter and extending through the raphe to the perineal integument. To complete the cure the patient must wear for a while a glass dilator.
Glass is better than any other material, because it is easily
kept clean, and its transparency enables us to see the cut surfaces and the vaginal walls without removing it. If there is
much bleeding the dilator should be introduced at once,
otherwise wait for twenty-four hours, when it may be tolerated
from one to four hours morning and afternoon, until the
parts are entirely healed and all sensitiveness removed.

. Some authors oppose this bloody operation of Sims' and
claim that this rebellious trouble can be cured by less severe
means. Scanzoni effects a cure by gradual dilatation; Simpson by dividing the nervus pudendus subcutaniously; Chor-
rier, Horwitz, Courtney, Sutigin, and Tilt by forcible dilatation under profound anæsthesia; and in America we have
even introduced "*etherial cohabitation;*" that is while the
wife is under the influence of an anæsthetic the husband per-

forms coitus with the view of inducing conception, and effecting a cure through parturition.

Partial or complete atresia vulvæ obstructs the entrance into the vagina and prevents conception. If the adhesions are so firm that the fingers or handle of the scalpel will not tear through them, we must use the knife and make an opening large enough to admit of connection.

Tumors of the vulva when so large as to interfere with or prevent sexual intercourse must be excised.

When with ruptured perineum we have sterility from an inability in the vagina to retain the semen, the defective part must be restored by the most improved method of operating for this class of cases. If metalic sutures are used and the operation properly performed, it is safe to affirm that success is the rule, and with this fact known, few women will be found willing to endure such loathsome trouble for years or perhaps a lifetime.

(2) *Obstructions within the Vagina.*—Cystic tumors and fibroids or mucous polypus attached to the vaginal walls, fibrous tumors within the walls, and fatty tumors in the recto-vaginal septum call for the intervention of surgical treatment. The fibrous and fatty tumors may be removed by excision, the fibroid and mucous polypi by the ecraseur or scissors; the cystic if pediculated, also by the ecraseur or scissors, but if sessile, it is better to dissect it from its attachment. When the cyst is only tapped and injected it will subsequently refill.

Atresia vaginæ forms an obstacle to the reception of the semen by causing intercourse to be difficult or impossible, and so leads to sterility. Whether the adhesion be incomplete or complete, the treatment is the same, viz: to restore the canal, if possible, and keep it open by the use of the glass dilator until the divided surfaces are covered with mucous membrane or until all tendency to contraction has disappeared.

Congenital absence of the vagina may be practically divided into two classes: 1. Absence of the vagina with signs of menstrual retention: 2. Absence of the vagina with no signs of menstrual retention. In the first class of cases operative measures are generally called for, while in the latter seldom or never; but if at all, only when, in a well-developed women, we are satisfied that the uterus and ovaries are pefect and that menstrual molimina have been present.

In some instances where the organs appear normal the vagina invariably expels the seminal fluid as soon as the penis is withdrawn, and not a particle ever gets into the uterus. In a careful physical examination of these cases we shall generally find a very short vagina, which seems sufficient to explain this peculiarity. The vagina being very elastic is put upon the stretch by the male organ impinging against Douglas' cul-de-sac, and when withdrawn the rectile force ejects all the deposit. No operation will make the vagina longer, and all we can do is to instruct the husband to introduce the penis to a depth proportionate to the length of the canal.

Fistulous openings into the vagina may cause sterility by permitting the semen to pass out through their openings or by a secretion poisonous to the spermatozoa. They should be closed by denuding their edges and bringing them together by silver sutures.

(3) *Obstructions at the Os Externum or within the Cervical Canal.*—It is safe to assert that obstruction at the os externum or of the cervical canal is the most frequent cause of sterility. It generally opposes the passage of the menstrual flow, and when its subjects enter upon married life other consequences are added which tend to prevent conception. These are congestion and inflammation of the uterus, ovarian irritation, menorrhagia, cervicitis, vaginitis, vaginismus, and dyspareunia. We do not intend to convey the idea that these consequences and sterility are always constant, but we do believe that where we have a narrow os or canal the latter will commonly follow. The association of sterility with this peculiar formation of the os uteri appears to have been recog-

nized from remote periods of medical history, and its revival
by the late Dr. Macintosh and others was only a recovered
legacy. Aetius points out the dependence of sterility on a
contracted os and describes the treatment of dilating by com-
pressed sponge tents. Its revival met with but little encour-
agement on the Continent, but was at once accepted by Prof.
Simpson, of Edinburgh, and Drs. Barnes and Oldham, of London, and is almost universally recognized in America. The
obstruction is generally at the os externum; but if at the os
internum, experience justifies us in the belief that it is commonly due to angulation from flexion of the body of the uterus
upon the neck, and seldom to contraction. If we forcibly
penetrate the occluded os externum with the sound, the point
usually enters into a sufficiently capacious cevical cavity, and
with proper manipulation passes through the os internum.
Of course it will not be claimed that because the sound can
be introduced semen may enter the uterus. We shall not explain the theories by means of which the semen passes from
the vagina to the uterus, but shall assume that the possibility
of meeting between the spermatozoa and the ovule is pre-
vented in exact proportion to the degree of obstruction existing in the canal or at its external orifice. The obstructions
may de classified in the following order:

1. The os or cervical canal may be abnormally small or
completely adherent. 2. The os or cervical canal may be
large enough, but the hypertrophied and hardened lips press
so firmly together that the semen can not enter the uterus.
3. Valvular closure of the os or cervical canal.

Cases included in the first and second classifications require similar treatment, and that the most successful is to incise the os and cervical canal. This operation was first performed by Prof. Simpson, and his method has been generally adopted, but some of our American gynecologists have
greatly modified it.

Dilatation of the cervix by tents, bougies, and metalic

sounds has been so unsatisfactory in the treatment of these forms of sterility that we should not continue their use, and clinical experience shows that incision is not only the most successful but less painful treatment and is followed by fewer complications The bad results occasionally met with are cellulitis, peritonitis, and hemorrhage.

Prof. Simpson used a one-bladed uterotome and divided the constriction and lips of the cervix bilaterally from within outwards, using no speculum and depending on his finger as a guide. With a speculum we can see what we are doing and the extent of the incisions. Greenhalgh, Martin Mathews, and Coghill have each devised uterotomes with two blades, but they are all complicated and fail to do their work perfectly, and the operation has to be completed with the scissors. An operation more effective and full of simplicity is that of Dr. Sims, who cuts only with the scissors and knife. His operation and that of Prof. Simpson are intended to accomplish the same purpose. Prof. Simpson operated in the dark; Dr. Sims brings the os into view. Prof. Simpson cuts from within outwards; Dr. Sims from the os externum to the uterine cavity. After introducing his speculum and bringing the cervix well into view, he divides it bilaterally with a strong pair of scissors nearly up to the vaginal attachment. If the os internum be contracted he then incises the tissues on each side up to the uterus, with his blunt-pointed knife, the blade of which being separate from the handle, can be inserted at any angle desired. In order to guard against excessive contraction from the healing process, authors introduce into the uterus bougies, sounds, dilators, and intrauterine stems, as suit their peculiar views; some recommending their use on the third or fourth day, others from the sixth to the tenth. The operation should be performed soon after the menstrual flow in order that the cut surfaces may be covered with mucous membrane by the next period.

Valvular closure of the os or canal may result from a congenital or acquired crescent-shaped os, or from some abnormal condition of one of the lips, causing it to overlap the mouth of the uterus. In the first instance we may remove the obstruction by dissecting out a triangular wedge-shaped piece, extending nearly to the os internum, and in the second by amputating that part of the cervix that causes the closure.

(4) *Obstructions from Malformation or Displacement of the Cervix.*—The infra-vaginal cervix descends into the vagina from one quarter to one third of an inch at an angle of of about 120°, with the os directed toward the posterior wall. It is truncated and has a diameter of about $\frac{3}{4}$ of an inch. As this represents the natural cervix, and that most favorable to conception, any other size, form, or position will prevent conception in proportion to the deviation from the normal. Conoidal and hyphertrophic elongation are causes of sterility and should be treated alike. A large number of cases tabulated by Sims shows a conoidal cervix in nearly eight-five % of natural steriliy, also that this peculiar formation is generally associated with a contracted os externum. That surgical treatment is sometimes successful in these cases we have practical proof in the experience of Simpson, Sims, Barnes, and others have thoroughly tested it. In defective development of the cervix but little can be done, and we shall only speak of those cases where it is elongated. The end to be attained is to reduce it to the proper size. Until recently the only means known to us for accomplishing this purpose was to melt it down with caustics, but this treatment is troublesome and protracted, and the results are never what we desire. A better method, which is simple and satisfactory, is to amputate. This was frequently done by Lisfranc. Huguier has recently brought it prominently before the profession in his amputation of the supra-vaginal elongation in procidentia, and the operation is now generally considered legitimate. The dangers attending it are few, death having oc-

curred but twice in ninety-one cases of Lisfranc, once with Sims, and not at all with Huguier. We must guard against opening the peritoneal cavity by cutting above the vaginal attachment, or wounding the bladder or rectum. The scissors is preferable to the knife, ecraseur, or galvanic cautery. In amputations with the ecraseur or cautery we have a large granulating sore that will require four or five weeks to heal, and there is always great tendency to contraction. With the ecraseur it is difficult to tell how much tissue will be included, and there is a probability of cutting through Douglas' cul-de-sac into the peritoneal cavity—a misfortune that happened to Sims when he was attempting to convince Prof. V. Mott that this instrument should be accepted as a valuale addition to uterine surgery. I do not object to the knife, but can see no superiority it possesses over the scissors, and severe hemorrhage is much more likely to follow its use. With either we can divide the cervix at any point we desire, and union by the first intention is obtained as readily after the use of one as of the other. The scissors should be strong and so curved at the point as to enable us to divide the tissues of the cervix evenly. Sims has invented an instrument which he calls the uterine guillotine. To obtain immediate union the edges of the mucous membrane should be united by two silver sutures on each side of the os.

Some authors, over anxious about keeping the os open, introduce tents into the uterus to complete the operation, but they interfere with union by the first intention and should not be used. If the os does become adherent it is easily divided; but the discharges from the uterus will most likely prevent its closure, and it will only be necessry to examine the patient within two weeks after the operation, and introduce the probe well between the lips, which may be repeated every week until all tendency to contraction disappears.

When the cervix is too large from chronic hyperplasia or hypertrophied induration, amputation not only diminishes its

length but promotes absorption more effectually than any
other treatment.

If a conoidal or elongated cervix is flexed from an uneven
development of the lips it should be amputated at a right
angle with the axis of the uterus, and the canal incised
bilaterally.

(5) *Obstructions from Displacements of the Uterus.*—
That displacement forms an obstruction to the entrance of
the spermatozoa into the uterus there can be no doubt. Of
505 sterile women 343 had anteversions or retroversions; the
anteversions predominating in natural sterility, the retroversions in the acquired. This great proportion of malpositions
could not exist did it not prevent conception. In displacements the position of the cervix is so changed that the semen
does not readily come in contact with the os, and if there is
flexion the angulation usually contracts the canal. We shall
deal with those malpositions only that fail to correct themselves, and shall present what we conceive to be the most scientific and successful treatment. They may be considered in
the following order: Anteversion, retroversion, anteflexion,
retroflexion, and procidentia. In anteversion, as in other
displacements, we should endeavor to replace the uterus, and
if possible retain it in position. The first step is so well understood that we shall speak only of the latter. The means
to accomplish this is by the use of a pessary or by shortening
the anterior wall of the vagina. As the object of our treatment consists in the removal of every obstacle to conception,
and as the displaced uterus, when not supported, ordinarily
falls into its unnatural relations, it necessarily follows that
we should use an instrument that can be worn during intercourse and will not oppose the transit of the semen. I am
acquainted with none that accomplishes this purpose so well
as the Hodge pessary or some of its modifications, In anteversions the one devised by Thomas, of New York City, is
the best. Its basis is a Hodge lever, but attached to the an-

terior aspect of this basis is a horse-shoe lever moving upon elastic joints; the curve of the horse-shoe rises up behind the symphysis pubis and lifts up the fundus uteri. Satisfactory results may be obtained by the use of this itstrument when carefully adapted to the case in hand.

Dr. Playfair has produced a modification of Thomas' pessary which consists in making the uterine arm of elastic watchspring, covered with rubber. The Hodge pessary or any of its modifications, when properly adjusted, interferes so little with intercourse that the husband may not know his wife is wearing one.

The idea of correcting anteversion by shortening the anterior wall of the vagina first suggested itself to Dr. Sims, whose success surpassed his expectation. This is accomplished by denuding two semi-lunar surfaces about one half inch wide nearly across the anterior wall of the vagina; one immediately in front of the cervix, the other, one or two inches below, as may be required. The surfaces should then be united as in the operation for vesico-vaginal fistula.

In retroversion we must depend entirely on the use of the pessary, and we shall find the Hodge-shaped instrument superior to any other. Pessaries never do good unless adapted to the individual case; for while vaginas have a general resemblance, no two are precisely alike, and an instrument that serves our purpose well with one patient may be positively injurious to an other. I believe that the indiscriminate selection of pessaries and ignorance of their mechanism are the principal causes of the opposition to them. The instrument must be adapted to the vagina with as much pains as are taken by the shoe-maker in fitting a shoe to the foot, otherwise it will cause uneasiness or pain and do positive harm. We are somtimes forced to try a dozen pessaries of different sizes and shapes to find one that suits, and for this reason I prefer, where the patient can remain under supervision, the blocktin, which is so ductile that it can be moulded at will. But

when she cannot remain under our immediate care it is better
to send the block-tin model to the instrument-maker to be
duplicated, in silver or vulcanite. They are not better, but
being less ductile will not lose their shape by the careless
handling of the patient.

If conception follows the use of the pessary it should be
worn until the uterus ascends above the superior strait, in order to prevent impaction and its inevitable result, abortion.
When inflammation has bound down the retroverted body of
the uterus there is greater danger of abortion, but pregnancy
and the gradual leverage of the pessary, I have reason to believe, may ultimately induce atrophy of the adhesions.

The treatment of versions is of course applicable to flex-
ions, but here the prime object is to bring the cervico-uterine
canal as nearly as we can into one axis, so as to afford free
communication between the cavity of the uterus and the vagina. The axis of the cervix may be temporarily brought
into coincidence with that of the body by the use of tents or
Wrights vulcanite stem, but it becomes flexed too soon for
conception to occur. Much better results may be obtained
from the bilateral division of the cervix, or from splitting up
the lowest incurved portion of the canal.

Procidentia is generally induced by hypertrophy of the uterus, elongation and enlargement of the cervix, or relaxation
and dilation of the vagina. When the displacement is the
result of enlargement of the infra-vaginal portion, amputation
will correct it; but if due to the other causes, all kinds of treatment are unsatisfactory, and we can not expect success except in the operation for narrowing the vagina just below the
cervix. This is done by scarifying the boundaries of a trow-
el-shaped surface about two inches long and two inches wide
at the base, the apex being at the urethra, and the shoulder
at the anterior cul-de-sac, in front of the cervix. The denu-
ded parts should then be united by silver sutures.

Vaginal or uterine inflammation and other abnormal conditions may produce a secretion so poisonous to the spermatozoa as to destroy all vitality before they can enter the uterus. The truth of this assertion is so fully demonstrated by the experiments of Sims alone that other evidence is unnecessay. We should remove the cause of these abnormal secretions by the various local applications, and conception will follow.

Just here I should remark that the semen should be deposited at the proper time, and that conception is more apt to occur just before or after menstruation. Impressed with the fact that sterility is usually due to an obstruction to the entrance of the semen into the uterus, many practitioners have tried the experiment of introducing it directly into the cavity by means of a syringe. Sims claims to have impregnated one women in this way.

In conclusion, let us remember that in sterility the fault is not always with the woman, and that it sometimes exists in the man from an inability to secrete living spermatozoa, or from some obstruction that prevents its ejaculation.—*From a Reprint of the Transactions of the Kentucky State Medical Society*, 1877.

The Cause of premature Mental Decay and Nervous Exhaustion Induced by Inebriety, and their Treatment.

By EDWARD C. MANN, M. D.,
Late Medical Superintendent N. Y. State Emigrant Insane Asylum and Medical Superintendent "Home for Nervous Invalids," 152d Street, Washington Heights New York City.

INEBRIETY as a disease—I might say with propriety an insanity—will never, in common with the other insanities, die out until the Anglo-Saxon race succeeds in producing, what it does not now produce, a physique and a brain capable of meeting successfully the demands that our climate and civilization make upon it. To do this requires a bringing up of tone of the physical condition of American women, so that the conformation of women shall be what it should be for the best propagation of the species, and that she shall have, what she has not to-day, the ability to furnish a suitable supply of wholesome nutriment for her offspring, as is the case with German, English, Scotch and Irish women. To-day the vital temperament is deficient in American women, and the nervous temperament is too predominant and too active, so much so, as to require an undue proportion of the nutrition of the body. Nothing is more certain than that the physical development of most of our American women differs very materially from the physiological standard upon which the true law of increase is based. The remedy for all this lies in your hands, gentlemen of the Association, in common with the rest of the profession, and it is to the subjects of diet, fresh air, sleep and tranquility of life of the young of the present generation, and to the general training of the young in educational institutions, that we must look for the production of a better type of physical development and mental stamina. I think that the influence of physical culture, especially applied to women, and its influence on the body, cannot be overrated, and that by due attention to this we shall see our young women graduating with health, with good muscular development, and an abundance of vitality stored up for the trying duties of maternity, and with the greatest possible harmony of action between the physical and mental organization, tending to good health, long life, and healthy progeny. Physiology points to the necessity among our American women for a better developed physical system, more evenly balanced in all its parts or organs, a greater harmony in the performance of all their functions, especially in reference to what may be termed the primary laws of nature, so that their children may not be weighed down in the struggle of existence with the curse of a defective organization, but be blest in the inheritance of a perfect anatomical and physiological structure in all parts and organs, with a resulting harmony in the performance of all their functions, with perfect mental and physical health and immunity from the host of nervous diseases that affect so large a proportion of our people. It may seem as if an undue amount of attention is spent in the consideration of this question, but having, by reason of my speciality, devoted much time in the study and investigation of hereditary disease, I am firmly impressed that, in order to eradicate inebriety and allied nervous diseases, and to check the increasing tendency to physical degeneracy among American people, we must aim at the extirpation of radical defects in physical organization. At present the average number of children to each American family is steadily decreasing with each generation, and the children that are born exhibit a want of vitality, a want of stamina in the constitution, and such a predominate tendency to physical degeneracy that threatens seriously, it seems to me, the perpetuity of our native stock. The pathology of the production of inebriety, in common with most other nervous diseases, consists, primarily, in an interference with the proper nutrition of the cerebal tissue of the fœtus, so that, even during embryonic life, the brain of the infant undergoes pathological changes which induce deficient moral power, mental weakness, and predisposition to the acquisition of all forms of nervous diseases, there being an ill-balanced and defective state of the whole central nervous system disposed to take on diseased action. These diseases would cease to exist if a true, healthy civilization prevailed; but inebriety, in common with other nervous diseases, owes its origin to an artificial type, from wrong habits, pernicious customs and fassions, and from an unnatural culture and refinement where the laws of health and life are altogether too much violated. These diseases have not been the growth of one generation, but of many, and by the laws of inheritance have become greatly increased and their effects intensified. To eradicate these evils, and to perpetuate the race as it should

be, there must be sound and healthy stock, and not organiza-
tions impregnated from their very origin with seeds of disease and premature decay.

We find in dipsomania the general symptoms of exhausted nervous power, viz: general debility of the body, inability
to walk even short distances without fatigue, general languor,
unwillingness to make any active exertion, great tendency to
sweat, more especially at night, but also induced during the
day by the sligtest exertion, and often an unsteady gait. I
have found these patients exceedingly prone to neuralgia.
the explanation of this is pobably due to the fact that there
exists in such cases a worn, irritable, hypersensitive condition
of the sensory nerve-cells of the central sensory tract, which
is the sole seat of true nervous sensibility. The central nervous system is affected beyond all doubt by excessive drinking,
and the degeneration thus produced I regard as a powerful
predisposer of neuralgia of the inveterate type. Aside from
the direct influence impressed on the nerve-centres, I
think that these irritable and hyper-sensitive conditions
of the central sensory tract is often induced by visceral
irritative disease of the stomach, kidneys, or liver, as frequently existing in inebriates, which almost necessarily affects the
sensory nerves which ramify in these organs, and from these
diseased nerves a more or less steady stream of irritative and
wearing nervous impressions is transmitted, practically without cessation, to certain parts of the sensory tract, to which
the sensory nerves from any given part may go, and, as a result, sooner or later the central sensory nerve-cells are brought
into that degree of nutritional disturbance which is the fundamental factor in neuralgia. The real seat of these severe
neuralgias, from which so many dipsomaniacs suffer, is rarely,
if ever, in the peripheral nerves of the affected region, but in
the central nervous apparatus. The heart's action is weak,
often irregular, accompanied by palpitation, and not unfre-
quently with symptoms of indigestion. A change has also

come over the man's mind, so that the very *morale* of the mind is changed. At one moment he may be very joyous and excitable, and then he will become greatly depressed. He will be very friendly, and anon very hostile. He will be so obstinate that nothing can overcome his determination, and at other times you may lead him like a child. The heretofore ever-ready and resolute man manifests marked indecision of character, and in other cases there may be an utter inability to fix the mind on any one subject, or follow up a train of thought consecutively. Any force to cause permanent intellectual activity must be mental, not a physical one. If the force be alcohol, which it often is, as it is becoming more and more the habit to resort to it for its temporary effects in this direction, the rate of interest paid for its use is frightful. Not alone is there a loss of tone in the character, and blunting of moral perceptions, but intellectual discrimination is much impaired, and impairment of all the mental faculties is almost inevitable.. The ideas are more spontaneous, less under the power of control, and any exertion requiring continuous mental effort soon becomes impossible. There can be no doubt that alteration of the brain is taking place *pari passu* with these alterations of character. It may be atrophy, or the circulation through the encephalon may be checked or impaired by ossification, or softening of the cerebral arteries, or some disease of the heart itself, or the neurine may be undergoing a change, particularly on its peripheral surface, as well as on the surface of its ventricles or cavities. The convolutions become paler, and the furrows shallower. The weight of the whole cerebrum and cerebellum is lighter and less complex. Softening of a very delicate nature, so delicate as only to be detected at post-mortem, by letting a little stream of water flow gently over the surface of the brain, may be taking place, or, what is very likely, and is often passed by unnoticed, because discernible only to a well practiced eye, which may not be present at the right moment for observing its attack, is a very slight fit of apoplexy and paralysis, so slight indeed that it occurs and passes away unnoticed and unperceived, and is recognized only in its after-consequences and permanent effects. From the date of such an occurrence, though loss of life does not ensue from it immediately, yet in its ultimate effects it is sooner or later fatal. The patient is an altered man, and never recovers himself. So delicate is the tracery of the nervous structure, that the damage of a single fibre, or a set of fibres, destroys the unity of the whole. There are generally three things present that lead to these attacks of cerebral hemorrhage, and as these attacks play a very important part in the production of premature mental decay in inebriates, it is desirable to thoroughly understand them and estimate their importance. The three things alluded to are: hypertrophy of the left ventricle of the heart, chronic disease of the kidneys, and finally degenerated cerebral arteries. The hypertrophy of the heart is a simple hypertrophy of the left ventricle, the wall of the ventricle being thickened without any dilatation, although in exceptional instances dilatation may ensue. The blood, in inebriety, is more or less noxious to the tissues, since it contains an alcoholic foreigner, and its passage into the capillaries is undoubtedly resisted by contraction of the small arteries, the vessels most rich in muscular tissue. The muscular coats of these vessels, therefore, are hypertrophied in antagonism to the heart. Since the small arteries are hypertrophied throughout the body, the obstructions, though each is slight, are in their sum total so large that in order that the circulation may be carried on efficiently, hypertrophy of the heart must ensue. There may be doubtless degenerative changes in the small arteries, so that there may be increased bulk with altered structue. It should not be assumed, I think, as it often is, that all the processes in the arteries leading to cerebral hemorrhage and apoplexy are of a degenerative origin, as there can be no reasonable doubt that the presence of alcohol sets up a condi-

tion of sub-inflammatory irritation which plays a very important part in the production of cerebral hemorrhage. The
sub-inflammatory irritation causes the arteries to lose much
of their elasticity, and become permanently wider, longer,
and more tortuous. This absence of elasticity of the larger arteries becomes, by the withdrawal of the aid to the circulation
in equalizing the flow of the blood, an important factor in leading to rupture of the smaller arteries. When the brain wastes
slowly, as it often does, the dilatation of the vessels, and the
increase in the quantity of the cerebro-spinal fluid, favor rupture very decidedly. There can be no doubt that the occurrence of cerebral hemorrhage in inebriates, resulting from abnormal strains, would be much more fequent were it not for
the provisions which nature has made for the protection of the
brain from suddenly increased afflux. The turns of the carotid and vertebral arteries, the free anastomosis of the circle of
Willis, and the small size of the arteries beyond that circle,
before they enter the brain substance, all tend to protect the
brain. The perivascular canals also exercise a protective influence over the vessels they surround, and in the corpus stri-
atum, where cerebral homorrhage is especially liable to occur
as its vessels are capillary in size, and proceeds from the mid-
dle cerebral artery, which is almost the continuation of the internal carotid, we find the perivaseular sheaths of very large
size. When I say, then, that I consider one of the principal
causes, if not *the* principal cause, of premature mental decay
occurring in inebriates, to be the occurrence of cerebral hemorrhage, or apoplexy, resulting from degeneration caused by
the poisonous effects of alcohol upon the tissues, I do not
think I overstate the actual facts. We generally have associated in such cases hypertrophy of the left ventricle of the
heart, as I have previously remarked, chronic disease of the
kidneys, and degenerated arteries. The strong left ventricle
and inelastic arteries combine to prevent the wave of blood
sent to the arteries from being properly equalized, and con-

sequently the smaller arteries of the brain, which are normally thinner than the arteries of other parts, and which are degenerated, receive the impulse from the heart's jerks, and being thus diseased and fragile—perhaps dilated and aneurismal—give way.

Before passing to the question of treatment I desire to briefly notice an interesting question, and one with which I propose to deal at length in the future. The question is that relating to the degree of moral or criminal responsibility which attaches to inebriates. Inebriety depends very frequently, as we well know, upon an abnormal organic development of the nervous system that has descended from generation to generation, gaining in intensity all the time. There must certainly be a modified resposibility when homicidal or suicidal acts are committed during periods of such abnormal cerebration. In such cases a criminal act may be committed in consequence of cerebro-mental disease without any apparent lesion of the perceptive and reasoning powers. In these cases also the mental disorder is of a sudden and transitory character, not preceded by any symptoms calculated to excite suspicion of insanity. It is a transitory mania, a sudden paroxysm, probably epileptiform in nature, in which convulsive activity is not reached except so far as the mind is concerned, without antecedent manifestations, the duration of the morbid state being short, and the cessation sudden. In these cases the criminal acts are generally monstrous, unpremeditated, motiveless, and entirely out of keeping with the previous character and habit of thought of the individual. Such attacks are transient in proportion to their violence. There is an instantaneous abeyance. I would by no means wish to be understood as advancing the plea that inebriety as a simple habit should exempt or protect a man from the consequence of criminal acts committed while under the influence of alcohol, but if he has unhappily inherited an abnormal organic development of the nervous system, so that mental delusion, weakness, or disease deprived him of the power of choice, and if we can say, but for the presence of those morbid conditions the habit never would have been formed, we should then look upon his inebriety as due to mental disease, and hold him responsible accordingly. If we in each individual case study up its psychological history, we shall always be enabled to come to some definite conclusion. For instance, in a given case, if I can prove to you that an inebriate who has committed some criminal act during one of his paroxysms has had a paternal or a maternal ancestor in an insane asylum, I certainly present to you a strong reason for pausing before you denounce the act as the simple outgrowth of a vicious habit. Again, if a man has committed a criminal act during a paroxysm of dipsomania which has appeared either in very early youth or in old age, after a long virtuous, and temperate life, or after a sudden mental shock, or sunstroke, I at once negative to your minds the hypothesis of habitual drunkenness. A very interesting case from a medico-legal point of view occurred a short time since, in which the writer was consulted as an expert. A murder was committed by a man under the influence of a small quantity of stimulants, which stimulus evidently induced a state of temporary insanity, or epileptiform attack. The integrity of the brain had been affected by a previous sunstroke, and the man had just recovered from quite a serious illness. It is well known that after a sunstroke a small quantity of liquor acts very violently upon the nervous system, and it might, therefore, be argued that he was responsible for the voluntary act by which he submitted himself to the influence of the intoxicating liquors. But the facts of the case were that previous to this time he had been accustomed to drink far more than upon this occasion with impunity, and had never before been intoxicated. This man was, therefore, in a morbid state produced by his sunstroke, subject thereby to a tendency to insanity, liable to be excited by intoxication, of which morbid state he was ignorant, hav-

ing had no reason from his past experience to believe that
such results were likely to proceed from intoxication, and with
no intention in his own mind to do more than take a very
small quantity of stimulus. As you will see in this case it
seemed the only proper way to hold this man responsible for
consequences which an ordinary understanding could recognize as likely to follow from immediate acts. I gave it as
my opinion that the murder, which I will presently describe,
was committed during a transitory state of moral epilepsy,
which was the result of a preceding sunstroke, the immediate exciting cause being an attack of illness, and the taking
of a small quantity of alcoholic stimulus. This state of "moral epilepsy" is a morbid affection of the mind-centres,
which destroys the healthty co-ordination of ideas, and occa-
sions a spasmodic or convulsive mental action. The will cannot always restrain, however it may strive to do so, a morbid
idea which has reached a convulsive activity, although there
may be all the while a clear conciousness of its morbid nature.
The case just alluded to had complained of pains in the head
and sleeplessness, which had displayed marked periodicity, and
which had been accompanied with great irritability of temper,
excited by trifles and seemingly unconnected with personal
antipathies. As has been previously stated, the person alluded to had been suffering from quite a severe illness, and after
taking a small quantity of alcoholic stimulus, went out to
walk. He met a friend with whom he had been familiar for
years, and a discussion arose as to the respective merits of
certain politicians, when, the discussion becoming excited, the
man drew a revolver and shot his friend. He then went, in a
dazed and confused state, and sat for some hours upon a river
dock, and subsequently went home, burst into tears, and informed his wife of the sad occurrence, and gave himself up at
the police station. There was no simulation of insanity by
pretending to be incoherent or by strange actions, and no attempt, either on the part of himself or his wife, to pretend

that the act was an insane one. There was, however a total blank in the prisoner's mind respecting the events immediately preceding the pistol shot, which shot seemed to have aroused his attention for the time, and he had no recollection of the fact that he sat on the dock for some time afterwards, as he was seen to do. Upon being consulted, as I have stated, I gave it as my opinion that there had existed, for months previous to the occurrence, a profound moral or affective derangement, which from its marked periodicity was evidently epileptiform in character, and that the sudden homicidal outburst supplied the interruption of the previously obscure attack of recurrent derangement. There had evidently been induced by the sunstroke in this case an epileptiform neurosis, which had been manifesting itself for months, chiefly by irritability, suspicion, moroseness, and perversion of character, with periodic exacerbations of excitement, all foreign to the man previous to the sunstroke. There are a great many cases among dipsomaniacs where, in an unconscious condition, persons can progress from odd or eccentric actions to deeds of violence, suicide, or murder, being unable to remember the circumstances afterwards, and therefore, irresponsible for their actions. The question as to the degree of mental responsibility attaching to such cases is one of great interest to psychologists and also to jurists, and one to which it is hoped in the future much more attention may be directed than in the past.

Treatment.—In the treatment of nervous exhaustion and premature mental decay, we should primarily direct our attention to the direction of the mental habits. We should endeavor to provide, constantly, easy and pleasant occupation of the mind, avoiding, equally, lazy inaction or violent excitement. We have in these cases to deal with a worn, irritable condition of the nervous system—an unstable condition, as regards its nutrition, its solidity, and its perfection of structure, which makes our task no light matter. We must be very careful that we make our patients sleep, or we shall have a preponderance of waste over repair that will balk all our efforts.   Our patients, by reason of the hereditary factor generally present, cannot, without great danger to themselves, do or endure what other patients might safely do.   It will be also necessary to supply the greatest amount of nutritive material to the brain and nervous system to repair the undoubtedly existing nutritive lesion.   We must quiet all abnormal nervous excitability and keep our patients calm and tranquil. Attention should be paid to maintaining an even temperature of the body.   Care should be paid to the condition of the excretory functions of the skin, kidneys, and bowels.   If there is headache and drowsiness, such diuretics as the liq. ammoniæ acetat. with sp. nitric ether are indicated.   Indian hemp has also proved itself in my hands a valuable adjunct in doses of $\frac{1}{4}$ gr. of the extract as required.   Free exposure, without fatigue, to the fresh air cannot too strongly be insisted upon.   One of the most valuable of remedial agents is phosphorus, which I always prescribe to be administered in cod-liver oil in doses from ,01 to ,09 of a grain after meals.   The cod-liver oil is one of the best nutritive remedies, as fat must be applied to the nutrition of the nervous system if this is to be maintained in its organic integrity.   The general effects of phosphorus are those of a stimulant, but it possesses a special power over the exhausted nervous system.   It is, perhaps, evanescent in its effects, but is never followed by a stage of depression which is noticeable.   It should never be ordered upon an empty stomach.   Quinine and strychnine are also very valuable as nerve tonics, and I have obtained excellent results from the use of a pill introduced to the profession by Dr. W. A Hammond, composed of phosphide of zinc and ext. nux vomica.   This I regard a specially valuable combination. When there is present insomnia, I am accustomed to rely on the use of prolonged warm baths given at bed time, conjoined, when necessary, with the use of the monobromide of camphor, in doses of from four to six grains. This is an admirable cerebral sedative.

I come finally to speak of the remedial agent which, in my opinion, far surpasses all others in its permanent effects, and which is comparatively little used. I refer to the judicious use of constant and induced currents of electricity. The essential difference in the action exerted upon the nervous system by the use of electricity, and that produced by drugs very often prescribed, is as follows: Many of the remedies commonly employed in the treatment of nervous diseases and in dipsomania for the purpose of restoring lost nerve force are *nerve stimulants* and not nerve tonics, in the proper sense of the term.

Electricity is a remedial agent which furnishes us with the means of modifying the nutritive condition of parts deeply situated, and of modifying the circulation to a greater extent, I think, than by any known agent. By the judicious emyloy- ment of the constant and induced currents, we have it in our power to hasten the process of nerve growth and nerve re- pair, and thereby hasten the acquisition of nerve power. The use of electricity does not, I think, act by contributing anything directly to the growth or repair of nerve tissue. Its action, it would seem most probable, is to stimulate and quick- en these processes on which the material and functional in- tegrity of the nervous system depends. The action of elec- tricity is always followed, in my practice, by an increase of strength and nerve force, and the results gained are gradual and permanent while the use of nerve stimulants has always seemed to me to primarily excite the nerve activities proper, and *not* the nutritive processes upon which the acquisition of power depends. The deceptive results obtained from the use of nerve stimulants depend upon the excitation of nerve activities and the resultant expenditure of nerve power, which is followed by a period of exhaustion varying in degree and duration. The careful and judicious employment of electricity

has always led in my hands to an increase of nervous energy,
while the employment of nerve stimulants has appeared to
me to lead, in many instances, ultimately to waste and diminution of nervous energy. In cases of dipsomania we have,
as I have already remarked, abnormal nervous excitability,
conjoined with cerebral exhaustion, and the two indications
which are urgent are, primarily, for increased rapidity and
effectiveness as regards the process of nerve nutrition, and
secondarily, to secure freedom from excitement and diminution of nerve activity, and thereby to check the waste of the
nerve structure and of power. These indications we can ful-
fil by the judicious use of electricity and nerve tonics more
certainly than by any other means, there being no other such
combined sedative, and refreshant to the central nervous system, and we can thus successfully meet all the indications in
cases of cerebral exhaustion and threatened mental disease,
except that of affording direct nutriment to the brain; which,
as I before stated, I endeavor to obtain by rest, cod-liver oil,
phosphorus, etc. The use of electricity seems to supply to
the system, in cases of inebriety, the stimulus which has been
withdrawn: as my patients have repeatedly told me that,
while under treatment, they experienced little if any of the
terrible feelings produced by its withdrawal under ordinary
circumstances. I have seen this so often that I advance it as
a scientific fact, and not as an untested theory. I have had
cases of years standing, who have assured me that the application of the electricity has been of more service to them than
anything they had previously tried. I have generally employed both currents, the constant and the induced, using the negative electrode at the lower end of the spine, or at the pit of
the stomach, while I applied the positive pole to the head,
cervital sympathetic, the cilio-spinal centre, or region over
and on either side of the seventh cervical vertebra, and up
and down the spine, making a seance of perhaps 15 or 20 minutes daily, and in some case twice a day.—*Medical Record.*

Editorial.

The *Catlin* again emerges from humble obscurity, to prune in the "professional vineyard." Its success in shielding the "tender branches" of society from the blight of empiricism will depend upon that measure of aid rendered by those members of the Profession who are able to contribute (that) necessary material to make the *Catlin* a destroying messenger to "professional ignorance," and also to make it an efficient medium through which, and by which, the State may be honored as well as all worthy co-laborers for advancement.

The many favorable notices of the press, as well as letters received from worthy members of the Profession, will strengthen and encourage us to still strive for that "higher standard," which "afflicted humanity" requires. Coming from those eminent in the Profession, will be remembered as pleasing recollections of our associations in the task of crushing out ignorance, and uniting the legitimate members of the profession into an organized body of educated intelligence, who may (then) deem it a pleasant task to labor for advancement in science, rather than for gain.

The bright expectations of the future of the profession, as well as for this feeble effort to aim for that "higher standard" so much needed, will only be disappointed or frustrated by a want of appreciation on the part of that profession, to fight the battles of which, the *Catlin* was conceived, and brought into existence. The proposed conflict will, by a united effort, be waged with vigorous decision, to the end that ere the closing days of another legislative session blends with the shades of the past, "professional ignorance and charlatanism" will have been consigned to that retreat to which such carcasess

belong. That this end may be certainly attained, the *Catlin*
will be yours,' *Gentlemen of the Profession*, as well as the
cause it advocates; receive, and nourish it in "infancy" that
it may with strength received from the profession, force irresponsible ignorance to seek other fields of "usefulness."

The (late) Legislature having adjourned its session without
reaching the proposed legislation to regulate the Practice of
Medicine, Surgery, &c., disappointing the friends of advancement, yet the cause has derived a certain strength, in a general awakening throughout the state which will assume such
proportions by the sitting of the next Assembly, as to compel a just recognition.

The measure, had many friends in the late assembly who
did all that was possible for its success; that they had able
opposition to contend with is evidenced by the failure. We
have no desire to censure the opposition for their action, knowing that time, and a united effort will remedy the evil, or en-
force the discharge of a (neglected) duty which was due from
that body to weak humanity found dangerously exposed. It
may be that the arguments of the secular press influenced
them in arriving at a wise conclusion, similar to that which
echoed from the late Session of the State Medical Society at
Des Moines:

"That the question of regulating the practice of Medicine,
Surgery, &c., is one which properly belongs to the people, and,
it should be left to them for its proper solution."

This wise declaration, without investigation would seem
plausible, but when contrasted with maxims in law as laid
down by Eminent Jurists, does it appear too attenuated for
this age, but it belongs to that age in which force reigned
supreme:

"As society organized for the better protection to individuals, the absolute rights of persons, were abridged to relative rights to them. For the rights surrendered they received a guarantee for security to life, liberty, and protection from harm to body, health, limbs, property and reputation; for which, they consented to be governed by a higher authority than individual, an authority embracing many individuals as factors to form government, the office of which is to administer for the best interest and welfare of the governed. Laws are enacted, the primary and principal objects of which, are Rights and Wrongs. Personal Rights pertain to individuals, and are such as may be acquired over objects or things unconnected with the person. Absolute Rights are such as appertain to particular men, merely as individuals or single persons, and belonging to them in a state of nature, which every person has a right to enjoy whether in or out of society; and they become relative (rights) when incident to persons as members of society standing in various relations to each other.

Wrongs, may be personal or civil injuries. Wrongs against general public rights affect the whole community, and are called crimes and misdemeanors. When wrongs are found to be detrimental to health, or destructive to life, good government will suppress them.

Liberty consists in the power to do whatever the laws permit, and which can only be secured by a general compliance with all orders and degrees of equitable rules of action, by which the weakest individual is protected from the oppressions of the strongest. That man should have the liberty to pursue his own substantial happiness, yet he should be so far restrained from that practice or conduct which may destroy the peace, or endanger the health or life of another. This being the foundation of law, demonstrating that certain actions tend to human happiness, and that certain other actions are destructive of human happiness, and which nature, right, and justice forbid.

Whenever human action is governed by intelligent reason, clear and perfect, unruffled by passion, unclouded by prejudice, or unimpaired by disease, laws restraining human conduct are not required; but when reason becomes corrupt, and the understanding full of ignorance and error, must authority be invoked to guard the vital interests of human health, life, and happiness.

The design and object of law is to ascertain what is just, honorable and expedient for society, whose only true and natural foundations are the wants and the fears of the individuals. Their sense of weakness and imperfections keep mankind together, that community should guard the rights of each member thereof, and in return for this protection, each individual should submit to the laws, without such submission on the part of all, it is impossible that protection can be certainly extended to any.

When society is formed, order of necessity will be preserved by authority reposed in persons whose perfections in wisdom, goodness, and power, by which they may discern; 1. The real interest of the community: 2. To endeavor always to pursue that real interest: 3. That the power and strength of character be sufficient to carry this knowledge and wisdom into action. These are the natural foundations of society; and these are the requisites which should be found in every well constituted government, the primcipal aim of which is to protect individuals in the enjoyment of their absolute rights."—*Extracts from Blackstone's Commentaries.*

The foregoing vital principals have existed for centuries: As truths, they will have perpetual expression in the spirit of successful government. A government founded on other principals than these is not worthy of intelligent recognition, and must perish because of its own weakness.

That the evil consequences of permitting ignorant persons to practice Medicine, Surgery, &c., is dangerous to health, and destructrive to life is apparrant.

Grave questions, in which good health, long life, and happiness for the people depend, should be referred to a tribunal whose qualifications and special fitness are such as will readily measure the attainments of "empirics;" We therefore deny "that the question is one properly belonging to the people, since they have not the special qualification necessary to determine the dangers to health and life.

PROCEEDINGS.

Des Moines Valley Medical Association, Reported for The "Iowa Catlin," By J. WILLIAMSON M. D., Secretary.

The Association met in regular annual session at Ottumwa, Jan. 16th., present N. Udell, of Centerville, in the chair. This Association embraces about one hundred members. Officers for the ensuing year are as follows. President, WM. M. Glenny, of Albia: Vice President, B. W. Searle, of Dahlonega: Permanent Sec. and Treas., J. Williamson, of Ottumwa: Asst. Sec., A. O. Williams, Ottumwa.

The customary routine business was transacted, and the following papers were read and discussed. Hygiene, by C. N. Udell; Dyphtheria, WM. M. Scott: The relation of Physicians to Social and Moral questions, by WM. M. Glenny; and Presidents Address.

The following brief synopsis of these papers is given:

President Udell took for his theme "The Culture of Beauty."

Every one whether cultivated or illiterate, is a devotee of beauty. Aristotle when asked why people like to spend much time with beautiful things replied, "That was a question for a blind man to ask." Much labor and money are expended to improve and beautify the mind, but how little thought is bestowed upon the question, how or by what means shall we bring our bodies to the highest possible perfection? A sound mind in a sound body, was an aphorism of ancient philosophy; body and mind, each was the complement of the other, and neither could be neglected without injury to the other. Great men usually have large, well formed bodies. Shakespeare, Bacon, and Webster were men of superb bodily development as well as massive brain. This law of course has exceptions. Medical talent should be enlisted in solving the question, "how can we bring our bodies to the greatest perfection?" All things rounded and smooth are pleasing to the eye, and the human figure should be the most beautiful thing in nature. Action and grace are associated with thought. Eloquence when not enforced by a good physique loses half its power. Strongly marked, expressive features are becoming in man. Features are formed in a great part by the affections. "The heart of man changeth his countenance" is a declaration to be found in an old book, not yet obsolete. The "human face divine" when not lighted up by intelligence and benevolent emotions has no charms.

The statue at Florence—*the venus de medici*—long the admiration of the world is five feet in height and thirty inches around the waist. The average american woman is two inches taller and only *twenty-four* inches around the waist. (The doctor then proceeded to give some general rules for the culture of personal beauty.)

Dr. Glenny's paper on the relation of physicians to social and moral questions was elaborate, and we can only touch a few salient points. It was an argument for a higher ethical standard in the medical profession:

Virtuous conduct is essential to the highest success in the practice of medicine. It was always so considered. The Hippocratic oath enjoined it. The immoral man cannot be a successful practitioner. Veracity is a virtue fundamental in character, but not all physicans possess it in an eminent degree. There is with many an every day yielding to temptation, an attempt to exalt themselves by exaggerated statements of the gravity of the disease that has been so speedily brought to an end by their superior wisdom and skill. Ignorant people are always afflicted with a passion for the heroic—the doctor in the *role* of an executioner, and the patient in that of a victim. Great things have been done, great things suffered. Such men never fail to beget strife and ill feeling in the medical brotherhood.

Intemperance is another vice to which too many physicians give way. The physician, charged as he is with important responsibilities should be at his best mentally and physically whenever called to an important duty. This he cannot be if he drinks even moderately. It blunts his perceptions, vitiates his reasoning, renders him awkward in his manipulations and liable to inflict serious injury. To make a man a drunkard through prescriptions for the cure of disease is a grave injury to the patient, but to become a drunkard himself and continue in the profession is to multiply the evil an hundred fold. Young men given to drink should not be encouraged to enter the profession. It is a question whether medical colleges should not reserve the right to revoke the degree in case the recipient become a drunkard. The country doctor is under peculiar temptations growing out of the fact that he is in the habit of compounding his own medicines, often when he is weary and feels the need of support. But Society is responsible in no small degree for the intemperance of physicians. Whoever heard a tea-table history of such an one that did not make drunkenness a trifling matter, and include an unmerited commendation: "Poor fellow; he had but one fault. He was the greatest physician that ever practiced in our community. We always felt safe in his hands when he was not too drunk. Indeed a few glasses seemed to sharpen him up, and he was all the better for it."

But we cannot follow the doctor further lest we take up too much space, neither can we at this time present anything of either Dr. Scott's or Dr. C. N. Udell's papers as we intended to do when we sat down to write.

AMERICAN MEDICAL ASSOCIATION.—The 21st. Annual Session will be held in the city of Buffalo, N. Y., on Tuesday, Wednesday, Thursday, and Friday, June 4, 5, 6, and 7, 1878. Rrepresentatives will be received from permanently organized County, District and State Societies, and also from the Department of the Army and Navy of the United States. A representation of one to every ten members will be received.

Books and Pamphlets Received.

The *Medical Record*, A Journal of Medicine and Surgery, for April 27., and May 4, 1878. GEORGE F. SHRADY, A. M. M. D., Editor, Published by WM. WOOD & CO., NEW YORK City.

———

The Western Lancet, A Monthly Journal of Medicine and Surgery, Edited by GEORGE HEWSTON, A. M. M. D., Professor of Theory and Practice of Medicine in the University of California, and JAMES SIMPSON, M. D., Professor of Materia Medica and Therapeutics in the University of California, Published by A. Roman & Company, San Francisco Cal.

———

Clinical Ginæcology, by W. H. WATHEN, M. D., Clinical Lecturer on Diseases of Women and Children, Louisville *Medical College;* Surgeon to Female Department Louisville City Hospital, Louisville, KY. A Reprint from the Jan. and Feb. Numbers *Richmond and Louisville Medical Journal*, also from same Author, *Sterility and its Treatment*, A Reprint from the Transactions of the *Kentucky State Medical Society*, 1877.

———

Press Notice.

The *Iowa Catlin* is the name of a monthly medical journal published in Osceola, Iowa. The first number appears April, 1878, and contains forty octavo pages, in which are some excellent selections. Dr. Edward Lawrence is the editor, and judging from his first effort in the present number is abundantly able to fill his chair.—*From N. Y. Medical Record, April* 27. 1878.

CPSIA information can be obtained
at www.ICGtesting.com
Printed in the USA
BVHW042007101118
532427BV00034B/484/P